THE PHYSICAL MANIFESTATION
OF SELF

THE PHYSICAL MANIFESTATION OF SELF

High Heels to Yoga Pants, with a side of IRONMAN

SUZ STOKES

35
DAY
DETOX

35 Day Detox Ltd

CONTENTS

*This book is dedicated to the greatest
teachers I could wish for:*

My Parents - Rex and Nancy Honnor

My Husband - Ken W. Stokes

"SOUL IS HAVING A HUMAN EXPERIENCE - MY BODY
AND MIND ARE THE RESULT OF THAT 50-YEAR
EXPERIMENT."

Suz Stokes

DISCLAIMER:

All information contained in this book is provided for informational purposes only. The book is not a medical book and as such is not intended to diagnose, treat, cure, or prevent any illnesses. Please seek further details from your medical practitioner for those areas that are of specific interest.

Contact email: suz@35daydetox.com
www.35daydetox.com

Thank you for your interest in my story

Over the past 10 years I have been on an incredible journey of personal transformation. The person at the start of the book is someone I barely recognise physically, emotionally, and mentally. Would I have her back. No way! I now have deep insights and a connection to my essence which has created a much calmer, healthier and happier person.

Have I done this the hard way? Maybe! But the truth is I did it my way. No easier way would have got me to where I am now. What is most important to me is that I never gave up. I took breaks and lost focus many times, but I never quit on the transformation process. And it continues to test and compel me in equal measure.

I see things now that didn't make sense before. For me the patterns were always present. I recall being told very early in my life that I had "helicopter" vison. The ability to hover over a situation and take in the whole. I'm intuitive, a virtue that has been invaluable, and has been put to good use in the last decade.

Writing this book has prompted me to decide to re-release the recipe book I wrote in 2014. Titled 35 Day Detox, Manifesting Change. It has stood the test of time and continues to be the major source of inspiration for healthy eating. For without a change in what we regularly consume we cannot change what we experience.

In sharing my story here, there may be parts that resonate with you. If so, you have my utmost compassion – for these are not easy times. I hope my views and understandings of the various situations are helpful. These will be helpful only insofar as you will see how I navigated my way through. Your way will be totally different as each of us takes the path that is most appropriate.

I adopted an experiential take on the nature of human evolution as opposed to a scientific approach. It is based on what I knew at the time – so by its nature will be flawed and limited – I have added perspectives with benefit of hindsight. That too will be flawed as it is missing what I don't know yet. On the flipside I have been in the unique position to see clients with similar stories, helping me further identify the repeating patterns.

My focus in this book is on the physical body. The cause and effect of our actions, the impact of emotions and thoughts. Missing is the dynamic of relationships – to do that justice requires a book of its own.

You can find the 35 Day Detox Challenge I created online at www.35daydetox.com, waiting for whenever you are ready. Life is the ultimate game, and we are being invited to play as if our lives depend on it. Because in the end they do.

With love and light,

Suz Stokes

2022

CHAPTER 1

Dubai 2011 - My first 10km run race

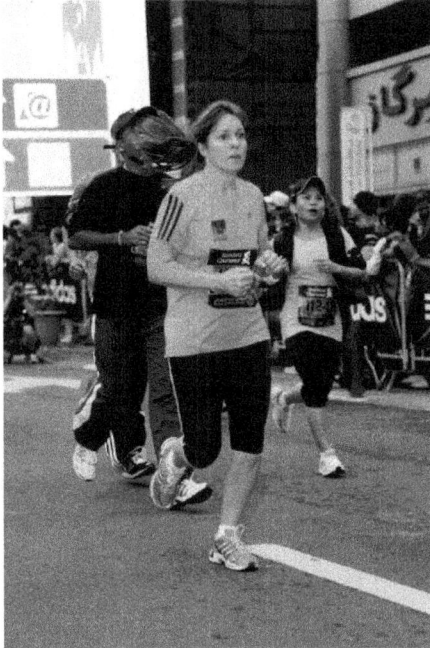

2011 was the year I turned 50 and the beginning of this saga. It isn't hard to pin-point the moment when the madness of endurance sports entered my life. Initially what I didn't see was the incredible journey of self-discovery I was embarking on. As I moved from my forties into my fifties, 2011 was the moment where I started to unravel the story of who I had become; identifying events and the experiences that had shaped my narrative, and most importantly learning who I truly was.

A confirmed non-athlete since childhood, it is questionable why anyone would include a 10km road race as a bucket-list item for that pivotal time. My other birthday requests for the year were more in keeping with who I was, including diamond hoop earrings, black patent Louboutin shoes, a holiday in Bali, and a party on a boat.

The answer cut deep into the core of the person I now was, and honestly, I was not very impressed with her, as I knew in my heart I was more than what my life had become. That feeling of the repressed potential had been glimpsed in my disappointment with myself a year earlier when I participated in my first sports event since school (the Wellington REAL women's duathlon) - more about that later.

For the 10km event I fronted the start line at the Standard Charter Dubai Marathon with over 20,000 people, including a few friends from the local fitness studio. Those friends were mostly ex-pat women from the UK, all younger and fitter than me, and after the starter gun went off, I didn't see them again that day. Among other things, I had not comprehended the size of the event. When the event ended, I was disorientated, it took me forever to get my bearings and collect my gear from the pick-up.

By then those friends had been home, showered, and were already congregating at the nearest alcohol-serving hotel. It was probably a good thing! Exhausted and emotionally drained I caught a taxi back to the apartment, crawled into bed (with clothes and shoes still on), cried my eyes out, and then slept for a couple of hours. When I woke, I thought it had all been a bad dream.

I called my husband Ken back in New Zealand and told him I had done it. We discussed the current state of the sales deal I was working on in the Middle East and what our dog Buster was up to. It was only January; the working year hadn't started yet but I was already fully in work-mode. This was the year I planned to retire; it was important to get a head-start on locking in business we had been working on for the past four years.

Nobody asked the details of the event in the following weeks, and I didn't say anything. All that mattered was that I did finish the run, and I had the medal to prove it. Time to put that moment of folly behind me and get back to my real life.

Amazingly I had even re-arranged my flights to be back in Dubai in time for the mid-January race. It would have been easy to have flown in a week or so later and enjoyed that New Zealand Summer/Christmas break a little longer. But no, there was a level of determination coming from within that was inexplicable.

Prior to turning up at the start line the longest distance I had managed was an 8km run/walk. That was only a couple weeks earlier when I dropped the car off in Paraparaumu for a service and thought it was a good training exercise to run home to Raumati South. My thinking was this way I was forced to cover the entire distance. I had my phone in case I needed to call Ken and be picked up. I ran 6kms before resorting to a mix of walking and jogging – a habit that would stay with me for years - even when it was no longer necessary.

* * *

Run training had started four months earlier with a "beginners running group" in Dubai. September was after the summer holiday months, the ex-pat community were arriving back from their home visits, and the weather was beginning to cool. The average temperatures range between a low of 30 degrees and a high during the day of 37 degrees Celsius. Humidity sits around 60%.

One thing I learnt from the early months in Dubai was that my face didn't sweat. After nearly 30 years of constantly wearing make-up and its daily chemical load, I had managed to shut down all the sweat follicles. That coupled with an inherited condition of rosacea meant that my face turned into a beetroot whenever I got hot, though it turned out that my knees were the opposite. Who knew sweaty kneecaps were a thing.

The fitness studio was on the ground floor of the apartment building in the Dubai Marina residential district. I walked past the entrance each day. If ever there was going be a time when I followed my mother's advice and did yoga this was going to be it. And in April the previous year I had joined the studio to start my yoga journey. The apartment complex also had a small gym, when I worked my way up to 3kms on the treadmill, I was proud of the achievement. In fact, on the back of that I probably thought I was now a "runner".

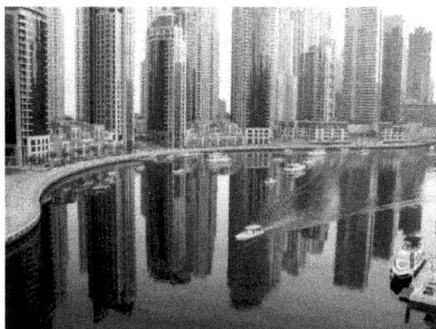

That first training run was to be an "easy evening run" around the Dubai Marina. The Marina surrounds a 3km canal of the Persian Gulf. The loop was bridge-to-bridge and approximately 7kms. The coach's pep talk indicated the plan was to go slow to ease the newbies in. I looked around and everyone seemed to know each other and looked like runners. Oops, maybe I was the newbie. When we stopped to stretch after the first 1.5kms I knew I was in trouble.

Frankly I should have turned around and gone home, but I continued. We crossed the road onto the incline of the overpass and to this day I have no recollection of the next 5kms as we wound past the Jumeriah Beach Residence restaurants. Apparently I walked the last kilometre home in the dark with the very concerned coach.

Back in the apartment building (and the air conditioning blasting at a near arctic level of chill), the lift doors closed, and I burst into tears. This might have been the first of the tears, but it wouldn't be the last time I ended up emotionally overwhelmed and sobbing. It was still over 35deg with 75% humidity at 8pm and I was delirious.

There was training again the following week – and I rocked up – I'm sure nobody could believe it. My humiliation continued over the following weeks because I was so slow. To compensate the coach sent me out before everyone else. They still all passed me – some circled back to chat – and then they carried on. Yet there I was putting one foot front in of the other. It would be a while before I heard the dubiously motivational comment: "You are better than those that are still on the couch"!

One of the studio's cross-fit trainers offered an additional Saturday morning training session focused on drills and general conditioning, and every few weeks the plan was to finish with a timed 1-mile sprint. For the record my mile pace was around 13 – 14 minutes, generally considered to be slow enough that you would be better off walking. Week after week I turned up. To the point it felt embarrassing – and clear to me that I didn't have much of a life.

Ken was back in New Zealand most of the time and I didn't have anything other than work and this training to focus on. It was only at my 50th birthday party that I finally introduced a partner who had almost seemed like a figment of my imagination for the past year.

Looking back, it is hard to fathom why I continued with this "interest". I wasn't good at running. In school I had a "note" to be excused due to recurring asthma and hay fever. That hay fever disappeared when I left home at 19. No one thought that I might be allergic to the cat (I literally woke up and sneezed every morning of my childhood).

The only time in my adult life that I had tried to run was a year or so after Ken and I got together. He had been a cross-country champion at school. We were on a holiday weekend away from our then home in Christchurch to Kaiteriteri in the Abel Tasman Park. Packing included me taking my knitting; he included multiple bottles of wine, a bottle of gin and one of scotch. Abel Tasman sits at the top of the South Island and has beautiful bays, and bush walks. At Ken's suggestion we attempted an early morning jog through the forest. I made it about 100m downhill before doubling up with an asthma attack. Soon afterwards I got an inhaler and we agreed that running just wasn't meant to be.

Within that kernel of complete running failure was a seed of my future. It was a part of my life that was such a no-go area that in the end I went there. If I had chosen anything else, it could easily have become a family endeavour. Also, I'm sure neither Ken nor I would have taken anything less than this seriously. It was a big enough goal to get our attention and I was prepared to move mountains to succeed.

Why? Because I just felt compelled to take that physical limitation out of my life. More than that though (at a sub-conscious level) it was also the fact of turning 50 and a realisation that I had never done anything truly for myself. Oh, I had purpose and plenty of successes and failures. For over 20 years my purpose was to hold together the company that Ken and I co-owned. My own personal measure of success and failure correlated to the current state of the business. And that ranged from successful to near bankrupt in repeating cycles.

Owning a company isn't easy and working with your partner is another level of challenging. I'm sure somewhere it is written that the combination is to be avoided in the interests of harmony and a happy life. Having said that, when we weren't concerned with the state of the company we had a great time, travelled extensively and were very close. Maybe too close, as for the first nine years we didn't have a night apart. Not many couples intertwine their lives so completely and in hindsight it was a major contributing factor to the level of stress I was living with.

Now 20 years later we were spending more time apart than together. This freedom opened an understanding that the communications security business we jointly owned wasn't an interest of mine – or more to the point – for me. The values of the industry didn't align with mine. Everything I was doing was always for others, or some greater good.

So this 10km race symbolised me doing something for myself, and when later that year I fronted to a Yoga Teacher Training (YTT) course, one of the first things we had to do was bring an item that represented who we were, or who we wanted to be. I spent forever wandering round the apartment wondering what I could take the following day. There were pictures of family and treasured items from others. In the end the 10km finisher medal was the only thing I could find that meant something deeply personal.

In Dubai the working week was currently Sunday to Thursday. As a Muslim country there are no bars or licensed cafes. Alcohol can only be served with a meal in a hotel. From this grew the "all you can eat; all you can drink buffet" concept. Nothing was more popular than gathering a group of friends for Friday brunch. For the ex-pat community, after a busy and stressful working week the weekend signalled dressing up in the latest fashion for a Brunch. It was a time to connect with friends and find some normalcy in a foreign environment - which basically meant drinking from midday. If it was a good Friday, the party moved from the hotel brunch to the Barasti Beach Club. Then on Saturday you could be sure that most of the 30 somethings from the UK would be absent from any fitness training or yoga sessions.

For me living in Dubai and the working week was a bit of an anomaly. I worked from home and the main objective of being in Dubai was to show a presence and commitment to the Middle East region. The reality was that I was occupying no-man's land. Present because I was likely to be flying elsewhere; particularly India, Southeast Asia as well as the some of the surrounding Middle Eastern countries. Engaged in multiple time zones as I was also juggling corporate activities in both New Zealand and Australia. In effect I lived a disconnected and isolated existence to maintain the multiple opportunities that Ken and I had chosen to pursue.

The evolution of communications technology was helping with my desire to stay connected. Now Skype was the preferred method of keeping in touch with New Zealand. Years earlier it was waking early in a foreign hotel to find a fax message slid under the door. Then it was traveling with two cellphones (one holding my New Zealand number and the second with a local SIM card). In order to maintain connection with my family I joined the social network of Facebook. And then it was only one slippery step before I was playing Zynga's Treasure Island with my nieces. With plenty of time on my hands it was very easy to invest time in something that was at best only a "virtual" reality.

Eventually one Saturday morning I turned up to the training and found I was the only person there. Everyone else had been at the 40th birthday of one of the women in the group the night before. I was mortified, partially because I had been excluded, but also the spotlight was on me training at something I clearly wasn't good at. It was time for me to be absent on Saturday too. Even if it was because all I'd done was go to the shopping malls by myself. Later it became obvious how much time I spent in malls as I could navigate my way round both the Dubai Mall and Mall of the Emirates in my sleep.

I don't regularly write in a diary, but I did have a habit of writing a journal whenever I got to the airport for a long-haul flight. Looking back at those entries as I write this it is a depressing litany of negativity. It does though indicate the first piece of the puzzle that triggered the changes that were to come. That of a failed business acquisition the previous year.

The final entry of one journal was from May 2011 as I returned to Dubai from New Zealand. Here it is summarised:

"As we wrap up the dramas that have been this chapter in my life. All comments previously about being out of cash pale compared to where we find ourselves at this point. The good news is that we have the deal I was working on.

Not getting to succeed with the (2010) acquisition has meant that we are no longer going to trade. So I am free to do something else after 20 years. I will have a party for my 50th/retirement.

My mantra is "I am complete. It is safe to use all my power to change now."

Before my birthday I am going to gather up all the broken pieces that is me and put them back together.

It didn't need to be this hard."

CHAPTER 2

Dubai 2011 - 200-hour Yoga Teacher Training (YTT)

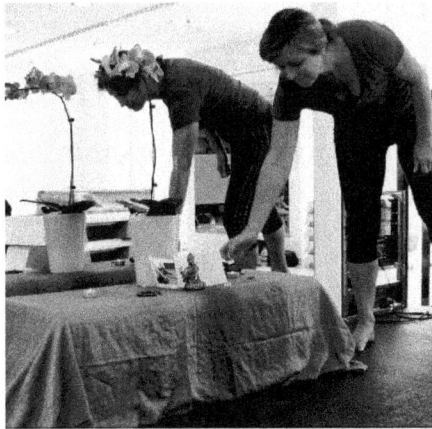

What a revelation!

Nobody tells you that Yoga Teacher Training (YTT) is a fast-track method of personal development. Throw a group of (primarily) women together for an extended period. They will all be looking for something more in their life. Some will have a vision of teaching yoga as their "Plan B". Challenge them to get out of their comfort zone on that yoga mat – and stuff is going to come up.

Most facilitators are equipped to handle the fallout – a few are not. Either way many of the people in the group are empaths. They want to help – they want to ease other's suffering - they often have similar experiences that are relevant. Cue the mini groups that form in the breaks and the deep conversations and connections that follow.

YTT is a pressure cooker experience, highlighting the various forms of pain and human suffering. Life is not easy for anyone and by the time we have reached adulthood we have been hurt many times. Physical pain comes from things such as injury, illness, disability, and poverty. Mental pain stems from grief, guilt, humiliation, and loneliness. These traumas form the basis of our limiting beliefs. Just as you will not wish to extend your shoulder past its current range of motion you will not willingly go back to situations that are flagged by experience as painful.

We have formed protective mechanisms that show up in our body, behaviours, and attitudes. All of this is exposed once we begin to practice yoga. Thankfully not all at once; we would be overwhelmed if that were so. It is often described like peeling the layers of an onion. Step by step whatever has been repressed comes up to be dealt with.

The famous Dalai Lama quote is very relevant as we begin to unpack our stories. "Pain is inevitable, suffering is optional."

Yet we are all stubborn about our limiting beliefs – otherwise they wouldn't be limiting, would they? We see them clearly in others – yet when it is turned back on ourselves it is very confronting. Cognitive dissonance comes into play here. It is a tool that we have developed that allows us to function within two competing beliefs. It allows us to hold a set narrative, regardless of what the real situation is.

* * *

At this point can I please say to those lovely souls who are still in my life, or who have been part of this timeline, there was nothing more you could have done. This is my journey, and my choice how it plays out. I know you would have offered more help if you had known, but you didn't know because I chose not to say anything. Like most people I have the capacity to pack away the traumas; for me it is generally by concealing a bigger trauma within the smaller. Being prepared to face and discuss the smaller while leaving the rest hidden. Sometimes burying them so deep that when hearing of another's experience, I empathise without recognising it is my story – until the lightbulb goes on – and I realise it is my story too.

This training module in 2011 was a little different in that it was non-residential. Rather than hanging out in India, or Bali, or another tropical paradise; for a month we were staying at home and convening in downtown Dubai every morning. Although going home provided a respite from the intensity of the yogic training, all the conflicting priorities of life remained and had to be factored in. My future trainings were residential and for me they were easier. In this post-pandemic world another option has emerged, that of the online training, that will have its own set of pros and cons.

It was a last-minute decision to join the YTT. Business in the Middle East was winding down for the summer, the family was coming to Dubai for my forthcoming 50th birthday and it didn't make sense to fly the 24 plus hours back home for a few weeks. Part of me probably concluded if I went back to New Zealand then there would be an excuse not to come back to Dubai during August, and I would not get my birthday party. The wounds over birthdays run deep within me. When my mother declared she was too busy at work to fly to Christchurch and celebrate my 30th I was gutted. Ken saw my pain and instead we flew to Greece on business and returned via Auckland to visit her and belatedly celebrate. Ken and I made the 40th a no-contest event and travelled to the US, celebrating in the Midwest.

I didn't own what I perceived as "yoga stuff". It took a couple of shopping trips and plenty of indecision to even buy the three-quarter sweatpants and t-shirts I thought would be deemed appropriate. Resistant to change is part of my by-line. I was born in the Chinese Year of the Ox. A few years later when I needed to buy a meditation cushion to take to a Bali yoga training, I hesitated so long that I ended up buying a cushion in Singapore's Changi airport. In my opinion that bright yellow candy coated chocolate brand cushion was ideal, and the best anti-conformity message to the yoga community.

Have you ever done a 90-minute workout in 30+ degrees Celcius in pure cotton? I was drenched, with everything sagging under the wet weight and there was still another 7 hours of the day ahead. Within the first few days the skin on my face literally burnt from the inside, crusted over, and then proceeded to peel away over the course of the first two weeks. Nobody mentioned how much of a toxic load I would sweat out for the next 5 years!

My only time of feeling like I was anything other than in the wrong place was one afternoon when I had excused myself that morning as I had to visit the Bank to submit some documents. Turning up in my high heels, dress, jacket, and full make-up was a shock to the group. Yet it was the confidence boost I needed. And to me, oh how far out of my comfort-zone could I get and still be showing up each day. From the initial 20 students who started the course we lost the one male after the first day, and one or two women left as the weeks went on. It is not for the fainthearted – yet like the genie in the bottle – once she is out it's hard to stuff her back in.

One afternoon it was time to all gather round and sit in a circle. This is the sacred circle. A space of connection and equality. Where you have the opportunity to be heard and to say what you may not normally say – both without judgement. To be authentic, to leave your ego at the door, and speak from the heart. Now all those years of censoring what you say to: not offend, fit in, compromise, will be challenged. By practicing non-judgment, you can be present – and learn to deal with being uncomfortable.

And then it was time to chant. I don't sing - not even in the shower. It was on that long list of things as a child that I learnt I was not good at. And we were just about to prove that even if you want to go beyond your conditioning it might take more than a bit of willpower.

I couldn't conceive of leaving the circle. So, chant we did. No problem, I can just look like I'm doing it. And then came the candle, it would be passed around and each of us would chant the next line of the mantra. All I had to say was "Shri Ram Jai Ram Jai Jai Ram". And all I did was squeak, my friend next to me is a great singer and she cracked up with laughter. "Suzanne why don't you try again," said the Teacher. I tried, more squeaking, and more laughter. Last try was a mistake on behalf of the teacher, the entire group was laughing and the point of chanting long since lost. I walked home that evening and wondered if I could catch a plane back to New Zealand after all. Surely this was not worth it.

On a brighter note was the afternoon where we had to teach the class something that was of interest to us personally. This I had no problem with. I had the perfect subject – how to arrange your life based on the lunar cycle. It was something I was passionate about, and a subject I knew thoroughly. By this stage it had been my experience for nearly 10 years. It would also be the fundamental principle that under-pins the 35 Day Detox Challenge that I later created. I might have been convinced about its relevancy but not everyone was. It rated alongside the presentation about how to set a table correctly using the various types of cutleries.

Did I mention about sitting eight hours a day for four weeks? My hips were so tight I couldn't comfortably cross my legs, and my core so weak that it was a struggle to maintain an upright position without using my arms for support.

As I said the practice of Yoga (and YTT) is not for the faint-hearted – it brings to the surface limitations and vulnerabilities. If you let it, it will be profoundly life changing.

CHAPTER 3

I'm healthy, aren't I?

At run training I joked that I didn't have a problem and couldn't put on weight. The usual topic of conversation in any gathering of people in pursuit of improved fitness is how to take weight off. Since I had changed my diet four years earlier, I had dropped 10kg and the scales rarely moved.

* * *

The trigger was at my 45th birthday I proposed that Ken and I go to a health retreat in Thailand. What I imagined to be 10 days of amazing salads and regular Thai massages turned into 10 days of free evening cocktails and lashings of self-loathing. It was the motivation I needed though and six weeks later I had stopped drinking alcohol completely. I also blacklisted gluten, dairy, and red meat. The bloating and brain fog disappeared, and I felt better.

It was more an elimination diet than anything as (over the next few years) each time I was stressed there would be another item I concluded I couldn't tolerate. They included all the nightshades (tomatoes, potatoes, peppers, and eggplants), any grains (except chickpeas and buckwheat), and most spices (including garlic, onion, and chilli).

* * *

By the time I rocked up at YTT I was subsisting on Chocolate Soy Protein Bars with a side of Chicken Biryani and Dal Makhani from the local takeaway. The concept of consuming healthy food had not occurred to me. All I knew was what I couldn't eat. And that list was getting longer year on year. I was using my mind to control my body, and that level of control was exhausting.

The saying "misery loves company" comes to mind. Which comes first? I was spending time alone in the apartment and cooking was something that I viewed as a chore and imposition. For over 20 years I had cooked every night. Takeaways and junk food were deemed unacceptable by Ken. Meat, vegetables, and ethnic cuisine choices were rotated so the same meal wasn't repeated within the month. I was excellent at distilling the meal options with my logical brain calculating whether it was chicken, Thai salad style over pork ribs with chilli beans. Each Sunday I developed the meal plan to by-pass the "what's for dinner" question. Nothing is more frustrating than both of us working the same hours in the same office and yet the expectation was that I singularly had the domestic situation under control.

On my own now I rebelled and reached for the sugary carbs to console a broken part of my soul, questioning continually how my life had got to this point. Later I would wonder if it was the other way round and whether it is the choice of food that eats away at your soul. At this point (and for many more years) sugar was the one thing I didn't considered to eliminate!

As a child I had eaten fresh vegetables from my parents and grand-parents' garden. The biggest treat was a glass of lemonade and "bought" biscuits at Nana's place. I followed this tradition in my Christchurch garden - even growing to like broad beans – as I had cultivated them my-self. There was no such thing as a microwave, firstly it wasn't invented and when it was then Ken was adamant that it nuked the food. It turns out he was right about that as the composition changes and is no longer recognised by the body as food.

Since being forced to sell our home in 1999 and alternating between apartments and overseas travel gardening hadn't been possible. My run-ning joke was that I had eaten enough vegetables growing up to never need them again. A little awkward when visiting India and its heavily vegetarian cuisine, but not enough to see the damage being done with my recent rebellious attitude to food.

Three weeks into the training and an education module on food to energise and heal was a revelation to me. There was an introduction to living/raw foods, enzymes, nutrition (macro and micro), juicing and cleansing, super foods, and the impact of food on mood. There weren't any experts available to instruct us and it was a brief dip rather than a deep dive. Nevertheless, the seed had been sown to radically change my perception of food and my health and wellbeing along with it.

Why didn't I know any of this? That weekend I went to the Mall of Emirates and purchased a Breville Juice Machine. In the local mini market I bought fruit and vegetables. In a fit of "healthy" I purchased a 750g bag of Chai seeds, used about 30 grams to make one chai pudding and left the rest in the cupboard. Six months later when I packed up the apartment to return to New Zealand, I ditched the lot. That was a step too far in my mind.

As the yoga course wrapped up, I joined Ken for a few days holiday in Bali. Thankfully it was not a repeat of my 45[th]birthday in Bangkok. I frequented the local massage kiosks beachside, purchased lovely cool cotton clothes and ate all my vegetables. I told the guest house upon check-in that I was vegetarian with a dairy and gluten intolerance. Rather than being a pain, the chef seemed to take it as a personal challenge. I would be lying if I didn't look longingly at the duck and seafood that Ken ate. And we did head to the odd restaurant at lunch for Gado Gado and Sate sticks. The strategy worked though and I went back to Dubai without having made myself sick.

* * *

A few weeks later I started checking out the self-help books in the bookstores. One book that jumped off the shelf was Dr Phil's "Self Matters". Not having owned a TV for the past 15 years I only vaguely knew of Dr Phil's television presence.

Self Matters was the tool I used to unpack a lot of the conditioning from my childhood. Throughout the 400 pages you are prompted to ask all the hard questions of yourself. What is important to you? Who were you before life got in the way? Where did you deviate from the core essence of Self? I was keen to get to the chapter at page 387 titled "sabotage". I knew there was going to be some gems in those exercises!

This was also the time that I decided to have a colonic. The concept of clearing out the large intestine with a water flush had been briefly discussed at the YTT. In some recess of my mind, I recalled Princess Diana had been a fan. I had read a bit about the potential benefits, which included improved digestion. And as someone with lifelong issues stemming from with digestion problems it felt like it could have been a piece of the puzzle. Instinctively I knew I was carrying a toxic load. There were risks associated with the procedure including a very interesting one about the likely emotional outburst afterwards. That made no sense until the following day I kicked off at one of my clients – uncharacteristically telling them what I thought of the incompetence we were dealing with. Oops.

During the colonic, without getting too graphic, the practitioner quipped that I didn't have a problem letting go but she did have a concern about how much undigested food was getting through my system. She recognised that I was in a state of chronic stress. At her suggestion I visited a counsellor/reiki healer within their practice. In brief; the reiki healer identified that I had a complete disconnect between my upper body and legs. There was no energy flow through any of the energy meridians between my stomach and hips - I had the blocked the first and second chakras completely. These energy substations are present throughout the body. There are seven major points within the body, and another five beyond the physical form. In addition, there are minor chakra points that can also be accessed for healing.

Any healing journey needs to start with first three chakras. Base/Root, Sacral, Solar Plexus. Energy rises and without the stability of the physical representations (body, emotions, and mental) we cannot interact with the world in an empowered way. The fourth Chakra is the Heart – and represents how we connect with the external world.

Put another way, they relate to our safety and security and right to express ourselves. Without these foundations there is an overwhelming sense of disconnect and being at the mercy of life itself.

This made sense to me, I had visited a Shaman some years earlier and he had said the same. That was on a 2004 business trip to New Delhi, India and our distributor had thought it would be a "something I would enjoy". The driver took me for over two hours through Delhi traffic to a private residence. It was very strange and dark, there was a lot of beating of drums and rattling of some instruments, and tut tutting about the state I was in. Most of it I didn't understand but I left with a scrap of paper with the following homework. I kept the paper in my passport holder for over 10 years before finally referring to it.

That homework was:

- Refer Intuitive Physician – Laura Koniver
- Download the Earthing Guidebook
- Tourmaline – grounding stone – grid your house

A piece of wisdom from the Shaman that I held on to was that I didn't fear death. That also resonated. Not that I'm in a hurry to get out of here, but equally I'm confident that this life is just one small piece of something much larger. I recall it was the first argument that Ken and I had. About a year into our relationship, I asked him why he was drinking so much, did he not want to be here, did he have a death-wish? And if so, could he please keep that to himself. These were the days before strict drink-driving laws and it was a potentially lethal combination to have a Tom Walkinshaw Racing V12 Jaguar on the road under the influence. His answer was that we were here, this was all there was, and when we were gone that was it. Usually I would have kept quiet to keep the peace, except on this subject I was adamant. I was sure there was more than the here and now.

The Shaman also said my spirit animal was the Bear, who had given up on me and left. I'm not sure that is the sort of positive reinforcement that is generally practiced in the West. I asked if there was any way back, there was a shrug of the shoulders and the suggestion that perhaps I could dance a little every day. I muttered under my breath: "Bye Bye Bear". That, singing and physical exercise were all part of the "can't do – will only make a fool of myself" stories I had been fed since childhood. At this point I still believed this to be my truth.

* * *

It was time to acknowledge the list of aliments I had decided to carry along with me at this point of the journey.

- Allergies
- Anxiety
- Asthma
- Depression
- Fatigue
- Gas & Bloating
- Headaches
- Indigestion
- Infertility
- Inflammation
- Joint Pain
- Skin problems
- Teeth grinding

It's a long list! These ailments had built up over time and were the physical manifestation of me. I didn't ever stop to ask if this was right, normal, or even acceptable. A bit like the hay fever that I didn't know was a problem until it was gone. This was a result of a slow and steady build-up of low-level poisons from that chronic stress into my system until it hovered right on the tipping point.

Interestingly the symptoms that bothered me the most were the ones I could see. The rest went into the category of "out of sight, out of mind." By now I just needed to look at a piece of chocolate to break out in acne.

* * *

If I was to sum up one core reason why I had got to this place. It was the enormous belief that I would sort myself out later. I would deal with everything externally with the justification that one day there would be time for me. Now I was turning 50 and, although I didn't know it, that moment had come. It was time to "pay the piper" as every action has consequences.

CHAPTER 4

Dubai 2012 - 17 hours of hell

The wheels of fate had turned and whether I wanted to retire at 50 or not that was exactly what was happening. For years I had said to Ken, "If I'm still doing this job at 50, please take me out and shoot me". I had seen too many ageing executives still traveling, attending trade shows etc., when all the enthusiasm for their role had long since gone. From my young and invincible perspective, the very soul of them was being sucked out. This seemed equally true of those in the corporate machine as well those outside doing it for themselves.

Now I was 50 and free. The party was over, my birthday year was over. What next? Christmas in Kāpiti loomed and then back to Dubai to pack up the apartment. There was no reason to stay in Dubai and even though the lease was expiring I had not given notice. I was not ready to come back to New Zealand, but I could not answer the question of what came next. These thoughts had been consuming me for months – jogging the Marina the conversation with myself inevitably came back to what did I want from life. I knew what I didn't want. I didn't want to be part of the industry we were in; I didn't want to work with Ken anymore, and I didn't want to live in New Zealand.

The reality was I didn't have an opinion, and without the conviction of what it was that I desired, I was stuck in limbo. I had no sense of self-empowerment; my life was based on what others chose. Though once I was given the direction, I was comfortable to move mountains to achieve the goal. It was the first step towards self that I lacked. All the way down to the smallest thing – my decision-making criteria was founded on a need to ensure I kept the peace - and if others were happy then I would be too.

* * *

I recalled a moment at the Rhodes train station in suburban Sydney a few years earlier. It was during the transition from Sydney to Dubai. I had packed up the Sydney apartment. Half the things were heading back to New Zealand and half were heading to Dubai. I stood on the platform and began to shake uncontrollably. What the hell had we done. The safety of New Zealand was still there but my life was going into the very scary and unfamiliar territory of the Middle East. It was daunting but deep down it felt right. This was my intuition at work, and from that space I had found the conviction to step into my power and make the move to Dubai happen.

Now a few years later that chapter was coming to an end. Had it been successful – or was it another missing opportunity – a opportunity in life that was ripe with potential that didn't quite manifest? Ken and I were picked up by the Emirates Chauffeur drive and delivered to the first-class check in. It was one of the rare occasions when we were travelling together. Not something I generally enjoyed as we had very different approaches to travelling. I liked quiet reflection time and people watching. He saw it as a time for socialising and meeting new friends.

Standing in the queue at immigration he went to one line and I to another – an act of defiance maybe. Not when he was through passport control, and I was on the receiving end of an official looking puzzled at his screen. Then the phone call to the supervisor, and the request to "step to one side please, madam". Then the "please have a seat in the office". Ken hovered in the background – slightly annoyed that we were not in the lounge already relaxing.

Apparently, there was a "hold on me leaving the country". The free trade zone had issued a notice that we had not finalised the release of the rental for office space. I was sure there were no outstanding payments. The lease hadn't been taken up as the 2010 acquisition of the company hadn't proceeded.

It was now getting close to time for the plane to Sydney to depart. The airline officials joined the discussion. "Would we be on the plane or not?" "Sir could travel but Madam could not", at least not until the release was provided. Ken considered it. Would he really leave me here to sort the mess out? Most probably, I had been doing that for years. My argument was that I needed someone to help me. We would need a lawyer and papers signed; he couldn't do that back in New Zealand.

It was serious, Ken left to retrieve our luggage and book the Meridien Hotel at the airport. Before he went, I pulled him to one side. If things went as bad as all the scary stories, then I was not prepared for what was about to transpire.

I took off my engagement and wedding rings, diamond hoop ear-rings and watch. I kept the Citrine ring and placed that on my ring finger. Citrine is a crystal of self-empowerment. All crystals amplify a specific area of the self and the yellow gold stone enhances confidence, mimicking the radiance of the Sun. And diamonds multiply the effect. The ring had been purchased on that messed-up trip to Bangkok in

2006. Back then I wore it on my left ring finger saying that I was getting used to the extra weight – ready for an actual engagement ring. Prior to moving to Dubai we had finally married.

Next, I swapped my high heels for flat shoes; luckily, I had a pair of Cole Haan flats in my handbag. Furthermore, I counted my lucky stars that I had comfortable and modest clothing on. I gave Ken my Dubai cell phone – he was going to be making the local calls not me.

Accompanied by the officials I was taken downstairs into the bowels of the airport and joined a group of a dozen or so other people who awaited a similar fate. What was that fate? We were loaded into two vans, one for males and the other for females – I was heading to the Dubai Women's Al-aweer Prison.

This part of the story has never been spoken about: Getting out of the van, being lined up, processed. Having my possessions taken from me. Seeing all the luggage piled in a corner. Hundreds of bags covered in dust. Inside was what nightmares are made of. I stood by the wall in shock. All the beds were occupied, there was nowhere to sit. I didn't make eye contact – I couldn't. After an hour or so a lady from Bali came over to talk to me. She asked if I would like to sit on her bed with her. She was chatting to others, and they gave me a brief explanation of what happened in the detention centre. Apparently, there was food at some point in the day, but I had missed it for the morning. I hadn't eaten – expecting to do so in the first-class lounge – but I was in no state to worry about food, or do anything.

Slowly the realisation came that this was my new existence. My possessions had been taken – I had no ability to do anything of my own free will. I had no choice of action; my only choice was how I would react to the situation. Eventually I lay down and closed my eyes. I didn't move, and I stayed like that for the rest of the day.

* * *

I thought about how at the YTT a few months earlier I had been confronted with the work of Byron Katie "Loving What Is". Of all the pre-requisite books we had to read – this was the only one I couldn't purchase as a paper copy. I had to listen to the audible version. I love to read, and I love to read fast. I will devour a book from cover to cover if I get the chance. But I didn't "love what is". I hated pretty much all my life. I had a very long list of complaints and injustices to call upon. It took 8 hours to read that book and then we discussed it at length. Finally, as part of the course graduation I wrote a report on it. As I had written that report my internal dialogue was "Wonderful! How can I love what I'm unhappy about"?

I had learned that the answer was acceptance. You don't have to enjoy where you are in life, but you do have to accept it, and find the appreciation within the situation. This forms a base line so you can move forward. Unless you can draw that line in the sand you will be on a repeating cycle of bringing the same experiences to you. How many times did Bryon Katie say to her clients "how do you know it is meant to be – because it is this way." Arrgh!

In all my time with clients of the 35 Day Detox this is the book I've referred people to the most, and the one I've loaned out almost continually. The other one is Dr Phil's "Self Matters". These two points - acceptance and self-inquiry are the starting point on any transformation process.

As I lay on the bunk, I assessed all the things I whined about. My biggest recurring complaint was that I was responsible for so much for others. Sometimes it seems easier to just do everything. You know that old story "if you want something done right then do it yourself", or another favourite "want something done, give it to a busy person". Over the years I had willingly taken on everything.

In the short space of a morning it had been traumatically pulled away. Now I was responsible for nothing. I had no rights; I had no ability to do anything. All those roles, as a wife, daughter, sister, business owner, and homeowner had all disappeared. The only responsibility left was for my own welfare. This was the stuff of bad movies and scary TV series.

* * *

Although I wasn't here for long, it would have major repercussions for many years to come, including physical, emotional, and psychological impact. It would take me through to 2019 to understand the true lesson of the situation.

***

Three years later I returned to Dubai and as I sat in the Emirates airport lounge, I wrote this:

"Words can't describe how relieved I am to clear immigration. In truth I knew it would be alright once I understood the lesson. The penny dropped yesterday when I saw that my prison is actually my life in New Zealand!

I'm still not sure whether I should have gone back – but then it did need to be done – and I've had little choice in the matter.

Maybe not 3 years' worth though.

Yes I did lose my way."

CHAPTER 5

Kāpiti 2013 - Kāpiti Women's Triathlon

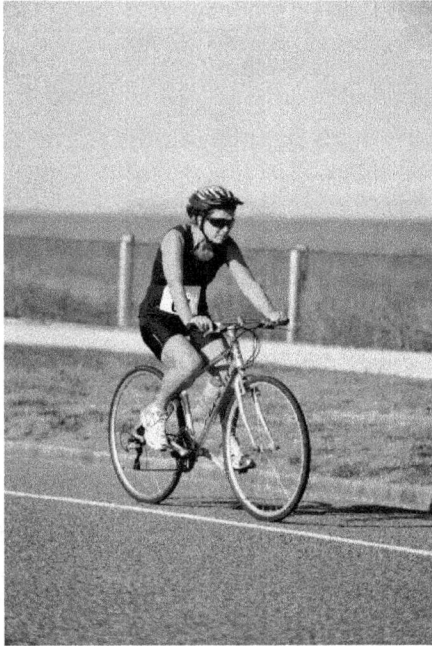

I was back in New Zealand, and resident on the Kāpiti Coast for the first time. I decided to make the best of a bad situation. I had found friendship in the running group in Dubai, and I planned to replicate this in New Zealand.

To me Kāpiti represents restriction and constriction. The very nature of the landscape mirrors this and the various communities are nestled along a narrow corridor of 40-kilometre coast between the hills and the seas. Within its boundaries a diversity of inhabitants has flourished. The retirees, families (often commuting for work to the capital Wellington), and an alternative lifestyle contingent. Kāpiti Island features prominently but remains out of reach. Drive north and feel the expansion of opportunity as the rolling hills and fertile plains of the Horowhenua come into view.

Kāpiti has an annual non-competitive women's triathlon – the Kāpiti Women's Triathlon (KWT). It has been operating since the mid-1980s. Hundreds of women of all ages and fitness rock up each February – KWT's motto is "inspire, motivate, and participate". Triathlon in general has a long history of association with New Zealand.

New Zealand has the honour of having the longest running international qualifying event that provides places to the Kona Ironman in Hawaii. Auckland hosted from 1985 to 1998 and since 1999 Taupō has been the host venue. The Ironman triathlon was conceived in 1977 as a test of multiple disciplines. Who would be the fittest? A swimmer, cyclist, or runner? The swim is 2.4 miles, bike 112 miles and run 26.2 miles. Almost all these events run with a cut-off time of midnight – i.e., 17 hours after the start gun goes at 7am.

Early in the year I wrote a very polite letter to the KWT coach requesting that I join her training group. I didn't receive a reply. Oh well that wasn't meant to be. Some months later I received the reply – training was starting in a few weeks, and she looked forward to meeting me.

Spring arrived and the triathlon training season had officially begun. Although the KWT wasn't until the end of the February the understanding was that the more training that took place before Christmas/New Year the better prepared we would be. A bit like that the belief that each hour of sleep before midnight is worth two after.

I still had a commuter bike from the 2010 Wellington duathlon. A duathlon general consists of a run, bike, run combination. The runs are short and fast, and it is all about the ability of the legs to adapt to the changing disciplines.

* * *

Now about that Wellington duathlon experience! In a moment of family comradery, I had bought a bike to double as an event bike (I only expected to do that single event) plus for gentle bike rides around the Kāpiti beach community. My first ride was to the Raumati Beach shops and back – 3kms each way – a grand total of 6kms. And that was the extent of the road training for the duathlon. I asked for a bike stand to be added. Hilarious when in later years it was all about doing anything to reduce the weight of the bike.

Regarding the event: the bike leg of the duathlon was out and back along the Wellington waterfront. I was going well, passing people, and generally feeling good. I hadn't appreciated that the first run of the duathlon serves as a great warm-up for the bike leg. All good until it came to turning around to come back. I had no idea of the need to change gears – so of course the chain came off the bike! No problem you would think – except it was more than 35 years since I had even thought about a bike chain. And I didn't have my glasses with me to see what I was doing. In a fog of frustration and near tears I fiddled with the chain. My hands were a blackened mess of oil and grit from the road as I considered that the best solution was to walk the 5kms back to transition. I would have to quietly pack up my things and wait to go home. Somehow in that moment the chain slipped into place, and I could continue. I was back on the bike, I was energised and passing a lot of the women I had passed before – and who had sailed passed me at the halfway point – my sister included.

Then on the final run, I ran out of steam and my only option was to walk – which meant everyone passed me yet again. I finished exhausted and defeated. Everything about the day had reinforced my beliefs about what I couldn't do, the natural order was maintained, and peace ensued.

* * *

November 17th arrived – the day for the first triathlon training – we were due to meet at the Paraparaumu Domain run track. There was light rain – I said to Ken, "Guess that will be cancelled, so no need to go". His reply was I had waited months for this – and I should at least go and say hello to the coach. To my shock training went ahead and running in the rain was apparently a thing!

In February 2013 I rocked up to the triathlon – no wetsuit, no clip shoes (in fact it would be a few races before they became a thing). I had a shortie wetsuit that was a couple of sizes too big. Why? Because in the shop I had no idea and didn't want to be a nuisance and ask for help.

After all the weeks of training I was prepared. Though not prepared for swimming with lots of others. I started to panic and couldn't breathe. In the end I resorted to backstroke, saving my tears for the bike leg, and run/walking to the finish line. For the first time I wasn't the slowest person.

I got a bit ahead of myself and later in the season and thought to turn-up at the Kāpiti Running and Triathlon 5kms race series. Now these are serious runners. I was back as the last to finish – again.

It was evident some of the women hadn't done the triathlon before, others had done it many times. After a few conversations it dawned on me that I had done it once earlier. As recently as 2011. In amongst everything else going on in the past two years I had overlooked that weekend. We had moved into our house at the end of 2009 and spectating at the 2010 KWT was proposed as a family outing. I had no idea what a triathlon was, wasn't interested, and on the day there was a tsunami warning, we thought it prudent to stay home; put the coffee on, open the bubbly, and fire up the barbeque instead. That should have been the end of the story – instead it was a seed sown, so when my sister saw that non-competitive Duathlon in Wellington the wheels of endurance sport participation were already turning.

Then the following year I came back from Dubai having completed the 10kms run. My sister and her family were staying in Kāpiti with us that week and her thought was to go down and do the half distance (200ms sea swim, 12kms bike, and 2kms run). I dusted off the bike, put my swimsuit on, and stood freezing on the start line.

My race strategy back in 2011: if I could get to the run leg without drama, I'd be fine. The reality was the water was freezing, and the waves were large. I panicked at the thought of swimming 50 metres out to the first buoy (it would be deep water), so turned with some others just past the breakers and swam along parallel to the shore. By the time I got to the second buoy I was so annoyed with myself that I swam out, took the turn and joined the others for the swim back onto the beach. I have no recollection of the rest of the race.

* * *

The benefit of training had become apparent to me. Triathlon wasn't a "hit or miss" affair where you rocked up to the start line and hoped for the best. There was strategy and a proven approach that worked.

This was the equivalent of my "aha" moment with approaching success in business. Richard Branson's quote "business is an endurance race" had inspired me in 2006 to take my physical health seriously in order to succeed financially. Now it was slowly dawning on me that I needed a strategy for my health and wellbeing if I was to live a better life.

CHAPTER 6

Being Authentic

Coming from a sales and account management corporate background it was very easy for me to see that stepping into the yoga teacher role could in fact grow to become a performance. Essentially you get up in front of a group of students and guide them through a 60 – 90 minute class, and as part of that physical session you are expected to impart some philosophy and words of wisdom. If the teacher hasn't embodied the yogic way of life, or understood the wisdom, then the message carries no deeper meaning and is easily lost. The best-case scenario is that the student intuitively recognises this and feels empowered to seek the lesson of the class within themselves.

In recent years the more dangerous outcome has come to light with many well-known yoga teachers. The inspiration a student feels in class is transferred to the presence of the teacher themselves. There was a possibility of putting on the perceived "yoga teacher" costume (in my mind yoga pants) and embarking on a life-style sales pitch – albeit in eco-friendly stretch activewear.

Within me there was a deep calling to not be that person. Over 20 years in the business community had left a massive hole in my soul.

When you say one thing and mean another it eats away at you. And this was particularly true of the industries and markets I had been part of. If I was going to teach yoga, then I had to lead from the heart. Back then I didn't understand what that meant. All I had was a long list of what I knew it was NOT.

Nothing is less authentic than the business environment I was leaving behind. Somewhere along the way it had become a game. One advantage of working in foreign countries is that when you don't understand the spoken language you need to learn to read the body language. This helped me see beyond the surface into the truth of what was happening on many occasions.

There was one time when we were in Egypt. I had arranged for the US manufacturer to be present at a top-level meeting. Our local distributor quickly concluded that he did not trust the manufacturer and on the back of that feeling he was not prepared to introduce them to his military client. Instead, he hatched an elaborate plan that included us presenting to one of his "friends" in another part of the compound instead. We went along with the farce.

Once we were back in New Zealand, we walked away from both the deal and the US manufacturer. A little closer to home was the time when I was representing an Australian company. They didn't hold out much hope for us winning a local deal - and when it became apparent that we would – they terminated the reseller agreement and went into the prospect directly. I would like to think in the 10 years I've been out of this world that the business ethics have improved.

Take that one step closer into the realms of personal development, from my perspective some of those self-help business books aren't about being a better person. They are about gaining an advantage in a situation, learning how to be something that you aren't, or somehow becoming more than you presently are, to get ahead in a career. But not just in the business environment, it's in relationships too. Most people don't like to say "no" – especially to your face – heaven forbid that you would be honest about how you feel.

The premise of yoga teaching is that you do not need to be an expert in the field to teach. You do however need to be on the path and be prepared to learn. For example, it is reasonable to teach the handstand pose if you are working towards it yourself. You may not be able to do a handstand, but you know the fundamentals. As you embark on your growth the appropriate students arrive and the teacher becomes the student.

To be authentic, it is necessary to be vulnerable. Vulnerability is not weakness; it takes more courage to stand as you are than to conform. Those protective mechanisms also serve to place a barrier between you and another. And people (especially children) sense when you are not speaking with authenticity.

Shield up, armour on, engage the defences. We do it all the time. And what are those shields; joking and laughter, bluster and bravado, deflection, to name a few. These are not conscious actions, they come from social conditioning. The mind likes to hold the status quo. Your inner critic will be backing you to continue behaviour that conforms. Ego is not vested in changing a situation, but the soul is.

From Wikipedia comes the definition of "Homeostatic": It is the steady state of internal, physical, and chemical conditions maintained by living systems. This sums up the mind's ultimate desire and the true opponent in the quest for personal improvement.

The Yoga teaching is that there is another voice within. That of the "observer", the one that is prepared to call you out, question everything, and (if you listen) deliver an alternative path. This can be called the higher self, true self, divine essence, soul or spirit.

When you consciously choose a path of self-inquiry and personal growth there is a need to master self-control. All physical, emotional, and mental responses are a reaction to vulnerability. Situations and people are going to come up to trigger the growth. Especially as those growth opportunities are being actively pursued.

With this in mind I embarked on a journey of yoga as a path for personal evolution. Rather than naming, recalling and analysing it (whatever it is) - it was going to be released on the mat. Alternatively I could have put my head in the sand and hoped the situation would go away on its own. Perhaps I thought I could settle into a new normal and get on with a life that was a close replication to what had been before. Not a chance!

CHAPTER 7

Napier 2013 - IronMāori Quarter Ironman

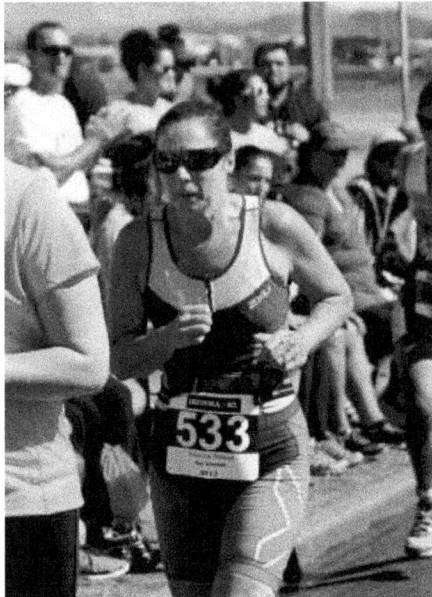

A few of us thought it would be great to continue to train over winter – we were enjoying the group training experience and we needed a new goal. Enter the Napier IronMāori. IronMāori was established in 2009 as a non-competitive event to encourage Māori to participate in endurance events, it is not restricted to those of Māori descent. The distance was longer than KWT but there is an inclusive vibe and an absence of cut-off times. This was the tribe I was looking for. We had a purpose. And I was a starter.

Napier is a beautiful town on the East Coast of the North Island. It was devastated by an earthquake in 1931 and rebuilt to the Art Deco style of the era. Members of my family lived there for some years, and I always enjoyed the vibe.

Ken took my new-found passion, or perhaps a better word would've been fury, seriously and gifted me a hot pink Avanti Questa for my birthday. That was in mid-August and by September there was a training plan in place. There were 12 weeks to race day.

My approach to training was diligent, and I took a cold hard look at what an endurance event truly meant. It was a very big hairy scary goal. And when the goal is big enough you will bring all the efforts to the table. Too small and it's easy to play safe and dabble. Although the Dubai 10km had been a massive goal it had not taken priority over work and family. The determination I had been able to muster was only enough to get me to the start line. Training hadn't got me to the end – adrenaline an a "I will not quit" attitude did. That might work for an hour or so, three plus hours was going to take more.

Now with my career all but over, and a large dose of righteous indignation as to where I found myself, I found motivation to train. Sometimes you need to get very angry with a situation to push through the inertia of change. This was my moment.

I knew I would self-sabotage in some way. My lack of belief in myself was interesting to say the least. Yet it was not that I felt I couldn't do it.

More that I wouldn't. In some warped mind-space I had equated trying with being something I didn't do. It was a behavioural pattern that would take many more endurance events to unpack.

At this point all I had to go on was the fact I had not "really" prepared for the Wellington Duathlon or the Dubai 10km run, and the result would be the same if I didn't change tactics. Yes I was likely to finish, but would I be proud of myself? Would I feel as if I had given it my all?

With less than six weeks to race day I gathered all I knew about myself and how I had been able to implement change in the past. I wrote out each of the dates/days and what I would ideally be doing in preparation. I set myself a 5-week Challenge to get myself into the best physical and mental space. Right here is the birthplace of the 35 Day Detox Challenge program.

* * *

Over the years I have frequently dealt with spirals of depression and anxiety. Depleting myself to the point where I become a walking shell with no energy, no motivation. There was a pattern as to how I recovered. I needed to tap back into that wisdom.

Often it entailed an overseas business trip. A time when I stepped out of my day-to-day existence and began to reclaim me. Sitting on a plane from New Zealand to Sydney/Singapore journaling and staring into space, walking into the hotel in drab clothes, booking myself in for a manicure, spending the day shopping in the CBD. Checking out of the hotel 24 hours later with a completely different perspective on life, ready to engage in the business meetings to come.

One surreal experience was flying from Christchurch to Sydney in 2007, only to find my bag hadn't made the plane. It could arrive 24 hours later. I was leaving for a 6-week trip in 22 hours' time. That trip included stops in Dubai, Abu Dhabi, Egypt, Jordan, Oman and The Hague. There was no way the bag would catch-up at any destination before I flew on again. All my work stuff was in the carry-on – everything else (including the luggage) needed to be purchased. My bag remained in Christchurch, flagged for collection upon return. When I finally arrived home I looked at who I had been and who I was and thought there was very little I wanted to keep. Those replacements were far more indicative of who I was at the end of the experience.

International travel was no longer the working plan of attack. Reflecting on these details led to the realisation that I could stay put and work myself into the best version of myself. What I needed was to clear some space physically and metaphorically. I cleared the kitchen bench and put the Breville Juice Fountain and Kenwood Smoothie2Go in prime position. Daily juices and smoothies were in. Food was fuel.

My favourite juice was Carrot, Orange and Ginger; I quickly learnt that not all vegetables and fruits go together. Some combinations causing very uncomfortable bloating. Years later I found charcoal tablets as means to quickly recover from my experiments. A safe bet for fruit was apple – it seems to go with most vegetables. Keeping like colours together created juices that were pleasing to the eye. Nothing worse than looking at a murky brown drink and trying to convince yourself you will enjoy it. I played around with mocktails too. These were great for family dinners. My pitcher of pina colada included the juice of a whole pineapple, coconut cream and fresh ginger. It was a particularly challenging evening when I made that mocktail and I ended up drinking most of it. The subsequent sugar rush was the equivalent to getting drunk and passing out. Job done.

* * *

My detailed training plan included - all the swim, bike, run sessions, the transition practices, sea swims and bike skills education. I was also armed with a weekly eating plan, yoga routines, and mindfulness practices to keep me "in the game". This was my first experience of becoming focused on achieving a goal that was internally manifested. To this point in my life all goals had come from external situations. The need to pass an exam at school, expectations of authority figures (parents and employers), or financial pressures.

We were prepared and on our way. But first we had to get to Napier. It made sense for me to offer to take my car. It was big enough for four women plus the four bikes – and Ken had his own car – so there would be no inconvenience. Only a slight problem. At this stage I had never actually put petrol in the car. In my defense, first there was no such things as self-service stations, and then I was living in Sydney and Dubai without a car, then Ken was taking my car to fill it whenever necessary. I had to confess quietly to one of the women and ask her to do it. I didn't bother to mention I hadn't driven outside the city limits in over 20 years. Seriously, I could fly to Saudi Arabia and conduct business on my own, but I couldn't even fill the car with petrol. It was another seven years before I realised those fuel hoses are retractable!

The distances were longer but there were no time restricted cut-offs. If I took my time, and maintained an even pace, it was doable. I didn't cry – but I did pee in my pants on the run – and there it was – initiated into the joys of triathlon. I say that with pride because it was the result of my commitment (mental strength) to continuing to run rather than stop and walk that last kilometre.

As we stood around chatting at the prize-giving we were all on a high from completing the event. None were more shocked than me when my name was called out as second in my age group. Even though I was happy with the day I knew I could do better – and you know what - I would do better. This was my first taste of manifesting a desire outcome from within and it felt great.

CHAPTER 8

Taupō 2013 - Half Ironman Team Event

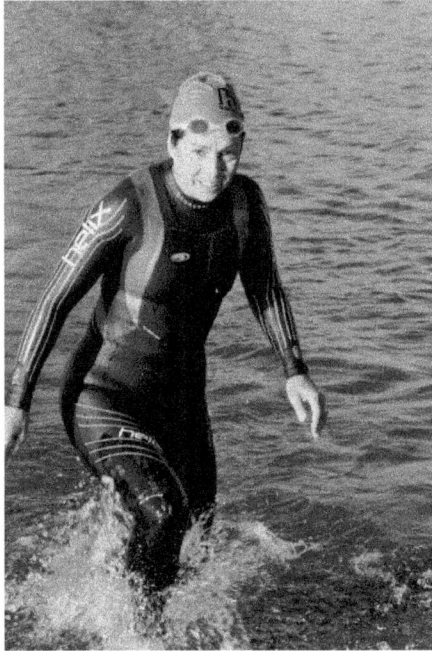

It was amazing to be away again with a group of women. The support and camaraderie were what I was seeking. Things were not great at home. I was resentful that I was back living in New Zealand. I envisaged that I would still be in Dubai. That door had shut. Living in Kāpiti was not what I wanted. Trouble was I still didn't know what I wanted.

We live in a world of instant gratification and expectations of a quick fix. I had returned to New Zealand, moved my focus from our business to personal wellbeing, and completed a long-distance endurance event. Surely the job was done and now I could move forward with my life. But life wasn't moving forward. In fact nothing seemed to have changed and with no immediate "crises" to engage with I was left in an uncomfortable void.

How better to see what this endurance stuff is all about that to do it as a team. Team events are a double-edged sword. On one side you no longer have the individual responsibility, it is shared. On the flip side is that your efforts count to someone else's experience of the day. You want to do well for your teammates.

Being a novice in such a professional event has its issues. Afterall Taupō is New Zealand's home of triathlon. Over 800 athletes came from around the country and overseas to compete. The Taupō swim was a mass start, it is very easy to get hit, swum over, cut off, sworn at - as men and women of all ages compete for the best position for the 1.8km out and back swim. My plan was to stay back, stay to the side, and stay out of trouble. Quite a few others had the same idea.

The reality was that I was not the slowest swimmer. Again I had trouble breathing – experiencing what I thought was a panic attack. Turning over onto my back was the answer (again) and a powerhouse of backstroke allowed me to pass other swimmers. It did not keep me straight though.

Forty-five minutes later I was out of the water and had tagged my teammate. It wasn't even breakfast time. Afterwards I thought – rather than being on the side-line for the rest of the day I could have continued and at least gone for a bike ride. Instead I grabbed a recovery breakfast and joined the others with cowbells, motivational signs and tinsel to make as much noise as possible as the cyclists and runners did their thing.

Watching others dig deep and achieve their goals is inspirational. Their energy is palpable and contagious. Yet it didn't lift me up, rather it highlighted what I was missing. The whole experience felt like an analogy for where I was at in my life.

Hold myself back, stay out of trouble, don't make a fuss, and ultimately side-line myself from the main event.

* * *

Still not to worry, I had the season of "distraction and excess" to contend with. Christmas was less than three weeks away and the extended family were coming to stay. Similar to birthdays the festive season had layers of stories built up over the years. From choices as to who would host, what food was served, and who was going to get the most drunk.

Mostly Ken would take out that honour. My attempts to limit wine consumption failed at the "only one bottle in the fridge at a time" rule as I was juggling two fridges full of food. When I opened the fridge door mid-meal and out rolled a bottle of white wine smashing across the entire kitchen floor I had two responses. The first was to teach my young nieces a couple of choice new words. The second was to log into the online classifieds website Trademe and buy a wine fridge. I was still sensitive to the fact for many years I wasn't deemed a suitable host as I didn't have children and therefore not a "proper family". Now that we had a house on the beach it was no longer a concern.

This year I was attempting to move beyond the traditional meat-based meals and had gone to some effort to create raw and vegetarian options. Nadia Lim's Vegan Roast Cranberry, Sage and Cashew Nut Stuffing Balls were such a success that by the time I sat down to serve myself they were all gone.

CHAPTER 9

Taupō 2014 - Kinloch Triathlon

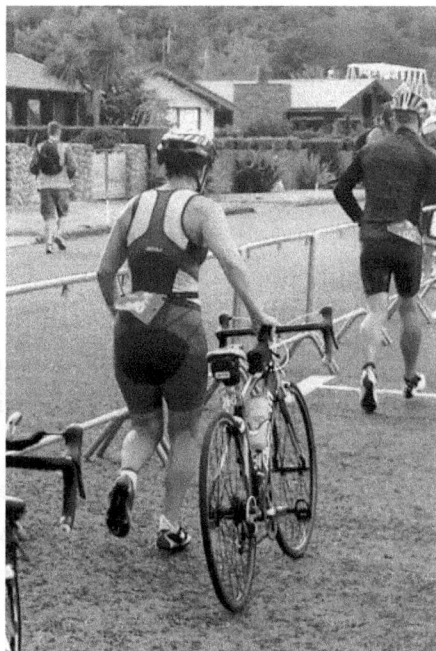

Having done so well at the IronMāori Napier Quarter and then fo-cused on the swim for Taupō, I made the rookie error of not taking the Kinloch triathlon as seriously as it deserved. Kinloch, on northerly shore of Lake Taupō, was the venue for the International Triathlon Union (ITU) official Sprint triathlon and part of the Sovereign Tri Series.

Triathlon is part of both the Ironman and World Triathlon brands. The distances are slightly different. No matter, it is still the Swim/Bike/Run format. I have a theory that it would be dangerous to have athletes on bikes or, heaven forbid, in the water at the end. Better that it's only feet and tarmac to contend with when physical exhaustion kicks in.

There were a lot more hills on the bike course than expected. Also, I had been lazy over Christmas, enjoying the summer and only training periodically. I guess in some twisted way I thought I would still have the fitness from the beginning of the season. The reality is that you may still have the muscles, but the conditioning goes very fast. I signed up for the Standard distance as it is about the same as a Quarter Ironman, i.e., just over three-hour (at my pace) event. We were swimming in Lake Taupō again – so no issues of salt and diesel (Pandora Pond in Napier) – and in February the water would be a warm 20 degrees Celsius.

Like much of life there is a very small window in either direction before we tip out of the comfort zone. Wetsuits provide warmth in the cold water as well as providing buoyancy. Without a strong core the ability to lift legs higher in the water stops the drag and allows a more effective kick. Triathlon rules allow wetsuits until the water temperature goes over 25 degrees Celsius, which was almost the case a couple of years later.

This was shaping up to be another cool weekend away with a lovely group of women. We hadn't managed to find one holiday home to accommodate us all (the group was rapidly growing) but we had adjoining properties. This, along with the lack of local hospitality venues, allowed us to pool resources and share quality time together. It had a similar vibe to my initial YTT experience. This time the personal development was being experienced individually and collectively as we faced our fears and tackled the triathlon course.

The swim started onshore with a small run into the lake and then we were off towards the first buoy. Turn right and swim to the next buoy and back to shore. Try and stand up, run for a few metres, and dive back in to do it all again. Jostling for position around the buoys is fraught. You are likely to get hit, kicked or cut-off as everyone compresses into the racing line. You can be sure I was the person taking a wide berth to avoid the melee.

Running to transition I was trying to keep moving and get my wetsuit partially off. All the while you are processing the shock of the adrenaline and having been effectively prone for the past half hour plus. A relatively good swimmer (compared to many triathletes who are strong in the bike and/or run), I was off on my bike in good time.

And then came all the real athletes.

There is a 10-metre passing rule. To avoid any advantage by riding close you are required to stay 10 metres apart. A rider needs to speed up and pass within a short time span, and then the passed rider needs to drop back to maintain the 10-metre gap. So here I was trying my best, being passed by everyone, and feeling like I needed to ease off to follow the rules. Who was kidding who? I just needed to keep plodding along otherwise I wouldn't make the distance within the time allocated. On that day I passed one person as we were going up one of the early hills, he passed me again on the flat, and that was it,

On the last big hill it was that hard going I thought it was time to get off the bike and walk. But I had clip shoes now and it wasn't even an option (I had seen it Napier but didn't think it would ever be me) – so now it was a question of staying on the bike. Pushing one leg down and then the other. My strategy was to count to 10, then count to 20, then count to 30, then count to 40, and then count to 50. And repeat. And I'd made it. Having cycled back into town it was necessary to slow down to go around the turnaround point. With so many faster riders converging at the roundabout it was a nightmare, until I realised that all the others were finishing their second lap and heading to the transition area to start the run. I, on the other hand had to negotiate the 360 degree turn and do another 20km lap.

* * *

By now the internal dialogue was working overtime and I was getting deep into some very uncomfortable thoughts. The season was ending, it was two years since I left Dubai. What did I have to show for it? What was I going to do now? I felt all this endurance stuff was a monumental distraction.

When I first met Ken I was following my father's footsteps as an accountant. By the age of 26 I was general manager of a computer bureau – looking after a staff of thirty. Ken's first decision when he acquired that company was to remove me from that role and offer me a position as CFO in the corporate office. The following year the consequence of our new (office) relationship was me being demoted into the role of a branch sales account manager. It's an understatement to say I had paid dearly for the relationship. Now I was blaming him for pulling me from Dubai too.

Once off the bike I was only able to run for the first 2kms before having to resort to a walk/run strategy for the remaining 8kms. The hill work had really taken a toll on my quad muscles, particularly the vastus medialis. Walking was what I expected – after all this was familiar territory.

* * *

What I couldn't see, or appreciate at the time, was that I was exactly where I was supposed to be. This lack of direction in my working life was my opportunity to sort my health and wellbeing out. I had been gifted TIME to focus on me. I was being shown via the endurance sports a way to MEASURE the progress along that journey. And I was thumbing my nose at it.

Something had to change. I had to change. Or more importantly my attitude needed to change. This "victim" stuff was not serving me. As I drove back to Kāpiti, I decided that Ken and I needed a meeting. It was time to put our cards on the table as to what were our individual priorities for the future. And from those two perspectives – agree a joint plan. Chinese New Year was upon us, the perfect time to reset personal goals. For the first time on my list was "teach yoga". Though I was hedging my bets as I also had "get a proper job" on the list.

I duly wrote my CV and approached a recruitment agency about finding a job. When the follow-up phone call came, I had a massive melt-down. Truth was I was in no fit state mentally to step back into an executive role. I felt broken and wondered if maybe I could get a casual job in the local juice bar instead.

Although I was reluctant to become a yoga teacher I was whole-heartedly committed to doing yoga for myself. I joined my mother at her local yoga class two mornings a week. My ego took a battering as the mid-morning classes attracted mostly retired women. I could not bring myself to join the after class sojourn to the local beachside café. Tuesday was a vinyasa flow class (exactly what I had been trained in), and Thursday was a slower restorative session. Both sessions helped me to find an equilibrium in the week. Vinyasa proving the energy and movement to shake off the lethargy and restorative helping me to become more aware of my present physical state of tension.

Each session always included a short rest at the end to allow the changes to fully integrate. Opening my eyes with that fresh view of the world was the highlight of my week!

CHAPTER 10

The Recipe Book

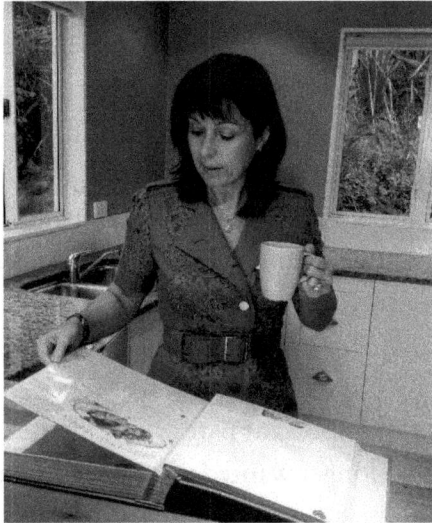

Since we had left Christchurch in the early-2000s I had been carrying a handmade recipe book from apartment to apartment. It featured all the classics from New Zealand's Cuisine Magazine. It is a mammoth example of scrapbooking. And an example of how I never do things by half. It also is an indication of how seriously I took the job of providing interesting meals on a daily basis – even if we were holed up for extended periods in places in the US such as Pasadena, Chicago, Minnesota, and Redwood City.

Over a period of months, I meticulously cut out each recipe and popped it into a contact photo-album. The project morphed and took on a life of its own. I started categorising the recipes in full. I added cut-outs of pictures, headings, and star-ratings. OCD and I are a thing. Finally I had to ditch duplicates, and if I wasn't sure which recipe was the better – I tried them both. Only when I was sure I was done did that magazine get consigned to the bin. That recipe book, plus my hand made tapestry cushions, were designated as the items to be collected in the event of an emergency evacuation.

The recipe book was referred to as the "blue-book". All cooking for over 10 years came from this book. It was the reference book as well as the inspiration for all our meals. Thanks to a recipe contributed by Annabelle Langbein it was a standing joke in the wider family that we were serving "possum fajitas" for dinner. Truly I had substituted chicken as the more acceptable meat that evening. When my sharp-eyed niece saw the recipe and asked her Dad what Opossum was, he replied "roadkill". What a great way to create a generation of vegetarians and vegans.

Food used to be an important part of my life. But it had become my living nightmare. I no longer wanted to go to restaurants as it was never about what I would like to eat. Rather it was a process of elimination. What will cause the least digestive upset, skin breakout, or emotional fallout?

The pressure of the corporate world was reducing. Days would go by without a phone call to take me to the brink. Emails could be dealt with slowly and in my time. Multiple times a day though was the question of what to eat. It may be asked innocently but the question was emotionally loaded by the time it was received. This time it wasn't so much about me cooking. Ken was preparing a lot of meals for us, however his approach was very linear. I was all about "substitute and work with what I had". He needed a specific recipe and all the ingredients ready before he would embark on any cooking. My vague, "replace this with that", and "leave out this, this and this" didn't go down well. Either I ate what was delivered or I did it myself. Now I wasn't prepared to go back to the former.

A great part of the human experience is the ability to enjoy food. What if there is nothing that you enjoy eating anymore? What is the point of life then? These were the type of questions I was asking myself.

There was only one thing to do, and that was to turn a negative into a positive. I had time in abundance, I could create the electronic equivalent of the blue-book. Incorporate the information I had received from the YTT into day-to-day life. Create a second book – this time with all the favourite recipes reworked so that I could enjoy them too. That way we would both be on the same page when it came to cooking. Researching online recipe book formats, I found a free publication app and started to cook my way through the book once again.

This time my recipes would all be gluten, dairy, and refined sugar free. They would feature ingredients that helped to heal the body. I wanted to go beyond the "substitute" route and re-imagine the way we put together recipes. I turned to the cuisines of other cultures (particularly my favourites of Middle Eastern, Japanese, and Indian), and sought out totally different ways to produce familiar foods. Freshly energised I got creative and turned the baking section into egg-free for good measure. For baking inspiration, I referred to New Zealand's favourite publication – the Edmonds Cookbook.

It was also time to create a vegetable garden. I had my eye on the unused lawn and clothesline beside the yoga studio. Even though it was a seaside property the large sand dune and ancient macrocarpa tree protected this area from the salt spray. I went one step further and declared that all new trees and shrubs had to be productive rather than ornamental. This was an investment in the future, and I planted and nurtured apple trees, fig, feijoa, banana, grape, blackcurrants and blueberries, lemon, lime, and avocado. The orange tree, tamarillo and passionfruit didn't survive. The jury is still out on the olives, pinenut and macadamia.

The biggest win I had was when I converted the family favourite "spag bol" into a vegan version using red lentils, and if mine was served on gluten free pasta with nutritional yeast it could've been a flashback to a meal at our favourite Friday night restaurant of the 1990s. This dish also became the comfort meal for the young HelpX travellers. I'm sure it is now being prepared in Europe, the US and South America, which makes me incredibly proud, and grateful to have aided in the saving of at least a few cows. The trick is to add finely chopped mushrooms (or Miso paste), to mimic the Unami taste of meat.

Not everyone is going to support your desire to change. This was a major frustration that I faced, and I know many of my clients have also faced. By producing the new blue-book I had eliminated the debate on whether a recipe was okay for me or not, and perhaps more importantly it was okay for us both.

CHAPTER 11

Kāpiti 2014 - Kāpiti Women's Triathlon (take 2)

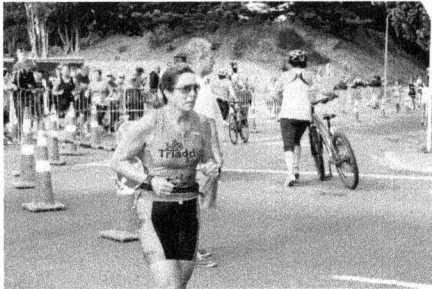

Now we did have all the gear and better still we had some idea. The KWT triathlon itself was drama-free. I had the proper wetsuit and bike. Training was consistent and the course familiar. We even had team kit and a shared picnic post-event. There was no expectation on time, though I couldn't help checking the results and seeing that at 1 hour 1 minute I was the fastest over-50 woman on the day.

The tribe had changed. We were all more experienced, our goals were changing, and the group was also changing. A friend wisely said that the people will change but the essence of the group remains. I wasn't so sure – I hoped so. But the reality was I too had changed. Whether the group dynamic changed or not I couldn't be objective about that.

Our training was getting more intense. We were doing long bike rides (over 2 hours), as well as going up into the hills surrounding Kāpiti. The group rides started easy with Mangaone South, progressed to the Maungakotukutuku Hill (elevation 360 metres) and finally the Akatarawa Hill climb (450 metres above sea level). It might have been hard going up but for me it was terrifying going down.

Often the conversation would go to food. Any sustained exercise over 90 minutes needs to be fuelled correctly. Otherwise, there is a "hit the wall", or "bonking" moment. Bonking is when the body runs out of stored glycogen. Instead of a breakfast of oats I was having a fully-loaded green smoothie. Something was working as I generally had enough energy for the morning's ride. My version always included a balance of carbs, protein, and fats. Carbs from fruit and leafy greens, protein from flaxseed or chia, and fats from avocado or coconut oil.

In addition, I systematically tried different combinations of whole food recipes to avoid protein bars and endurance gels. Avoiding chemicals was important to me (and my sensitive digestive system). I had previously tried a gel on a training run. Let's just say that the advice to test them - while knowing the location of the next public toilet - is valid.

What I did know was that after many years of knowingly and unknowingly abusing my digestive system I was walking a very fine line in terms of nutrition. And if I got it even slightly wrong then I would not be able to cope with the intensity of the training sessions. Having decided to do endurance events this was sufficient motivation to make the hard food and drink choices.

On one bike ride the conversation was about losing weight as well as training. I innocently piped up that I thought what I was doing had some relevance. Oops, I was put in my place very quickly and firmly told that I wasn't over-weight and therefore I should keep my thoughts to myself. Well I really did think I had something to contribute to the conversation. So I quietly said to the recipient of the well-meaning advice, "I will give you some of my recipes to try." Nothing like a bit of outside pressure to keep me honest in the development of the new blue-book.

The first week was easy as I had already done the smoothies for the breakfast section. How hard can it be to maintain a "half-dozen recipes per week" pace for five weeks? i.e. Breakfast, Snacks, Lunch, Dinner and Desserts. Truth was it was very difficult as each week I needed to focus on those meals, try the recipe, photograph the results, check out the nutritional profile and write and print the final ingredient list and instructions. And not all efforts were successful! Still when I start something I have the stubbornness of my Chinese Horoscope Ox to continue. It was finally time to wrap up the project when there was over 100 recipes and 165 pages in the new "blue-book".

Each week I would surreptitiously roll printed pages of recipes and place them in an empty drink bottle on my bike. At the end of the ride, I would hand them over to my friend. As the queries came in, I realised that an important part of the puzzle was missing. There needed to be an accompanying explanation that answered the WHY as well as some of the other things that I was doing to support the detox process. It wasn't just the food that makes a difference to the body. And that is how the "tips & tricks" section of the book came about. A year later this section was lifted from the recipe book to form the foundation of the 5-week detox challenge.

* * *

I would like to say I embraced this new life whole-heartedly but that is far from the truth. I was very angry that I was "in retirement" on the Kāpiti Coast. Although I was happy to be out of our business, I didn't think I would be side-lined completely from a corporate career. I liked feeling better because of the good nutritious food but a part of me just wanted to be a normal unhealthy person like others. From my perspective it looked like a much easier option.

There is a seductive energy about the familiar, the rules and rituals that we abide by. Those that keep us within a narrow band of behaviour. Even if the constraints have unpleasant consequences, we often prefer them to the unfamiliar. Boundaries give the illusion of control. And a feeling of control is more comforting than acknowledging that life is inherently out of our control.

Honestly, even though I had been incredibly unhealthy I enjoyed my life. Up until about age 45 it was fun. I met interesting people, stayed at amazing hotels, and clocked up over 900,000 flight miles with Emirates airline alone. I missed the excitement of travelling internationally and working on big deals. Of putting on business clothes and being valued accordingly. Things had changed, I had changed internally, now my external world was changing too.

Slowly I started to donate the clothes, handbags, and shoes to charity. As the months wore on, I could see that even if I did get back into the corporate world, I wouldn't want to wear the same things. I gathered up the formal evening clothes and donated them too. One trick I learnt along the way was when something is really hard to let go of – it helps to take a photo as a memento – then it can be easier to let the actual item depart gracefully.

The packing boxes from Dubai filled an entire garage, where they remained for another six months (over two years in total) before we finally sold the furniture and artwork that didn't belong in a beach-house. We had been down this track before, putting our furniture etc. in storage in 1999 and only bringing it out in 2006. Back then I was so confident that we would be settled in a new place within six months I had asked the moving company to temporarily look after dozens of pot plants.

Now all that remained was the business paraphernalia – it was like a festering sore – resolved by ordering a skip and dumping the contents. Of course, the Universe had the last laugh (or was it a test) as within days a long-standing client sent an order for some replacement units and parts. I wrote back reminding them that we had advised that the product was at "end of life" over 18 months earlier. It was the first time I hadn't tried to "fix" the situation, although I did suggest they contact the US distributor to see if they had what was needed. Turned out they were both playing outside their territory for a random African deal – I was so pleased to be out of the loop.

* * *

I may not have been able to get a "job" but I could teach yoga. Ken had recently rebuilt the original shed into a yoga studio with the hopes that I would find the motivation to pursue this new direction. My view was that it was "very unlikely", and I would not be so easily pacified. Still, the studio was sitting empty on the property and all I needed to do was invite some of my triathlete buddies to join me. Firstly though I started some sessions at the park and on the beach (sunset yoga was a hit even in winter) before finally conceding that he was right.

It says a lot about my lack of confidence in that I suggested a "gold coin" donation for attendance. Gone were the days of negotiating multi-million dollar deals with foreign government clients.

CHAPTER 12

Wellington 2014 - Half Marathon

My sister was doing her first full marathon. Where I had gone down the triathlon route, she had chosen to run a marathon as her goal. I wanted to go with the rest of the family and support her. Why not do a half marathon while I was there.

I had done the half marathon distance at Waiterere the previous year. That was a two-loop track through the forest – stunning – except when it had been raining for a few days and it was over 2 hours of playing "miss the puddles", and "stay on your feet". Waiterere Beach Forest has another claim to fame as the location for a scene in the Lord of the Rings movie - think Osgiliath Wood to appreciate my first opportunity to run in the spectacular New Zealand wilderness.

At the 17km mark of the Wellington Half I pulled up and started to walk. The course goes out from the Stadium, following the road around the bays towards the airport and returns. On the way back it cuts in to take the runners along the waterfront. It is a flat course, with the wind bouncing around so much that you feel like you are always running into it. Once back on the harbour boardwalk I was following the same path as the 2010 Duathlon, albeit in reverse. All those feelings came back. Why was I doing this? Was it necessary? I just didn't see the point of pushing myself. I was expecting to walk. Although all the training suggested it wouldn't be necessary. The more I did the walk/run in those last few kilometres the more I told myself it was OK. Even when I could see the pace was slowing down significantly.

I began to get interested in why I was stopping to walk so consistently. It happened in training as well as races. This eventually led me to the 2013 book by Sakyong Mipham "Running with the Mind of Meditation: Lessons for Training Body and Mind". Sakyong Mipham is a Tibetan lama and leader of Shambhala, who has an interest in running. He espouses a theory of 5 stages of running equating to 5 stages of their meditation principles (Tiger, Lion, Garuda, Dragon, Windhorse). At the Tiger phase you develop the physical ability to run by concentrating on learning running and breathing techniques and building the required stamina. The next stage (Lion) will be taming the mind; no longer focused on the effort of running the mind needs to be directed elsewhere. Ideally into the present moment, appreciating the scenery and with awareness of the breath and body.

For now, all I could say was that each time I got exhausted I would begin to think about problems in my life. And the moment I started to think of those problems I would be so overwhelmed with negative thoughts that walking seemed to be the least of my worries.

It was time to deal with the "elephant in the room". Being a doormat was not helping me, quite the contrary it was a major cause of stress. I had blamed my stress on work and travelling – but when the work diminished the stress remained. Knowingly eating foods that caused me problems, holding back from saying how I felt, and constantly modifying my behaviour to keep the peace. These were my patterns learnt from childhood. Time to admit that I was in the grips of a narcissistic mother. This was the question I posed of myself: How can I show up as an authentic yoga teacher when I am not being authentic in my family relationships?

* * *

Two major moments of fate occurred in conjunction with this event. The wheel of destiny had turned yet again.

The next day my mother called and asked me to take her to see a dog at the SPCA. She had been looking for a companion dog for some time and the shelter had called her with news of a possible match. I really wanted to rest and go later in the week but she was concerned that a little corgi terrier cross called Jojo would be gone by then. I acquiesced and we went to the kennels.

It broke my heart to see the dogs there. And Jojo was so stressed she pee'd in the hallway. Ominously the manager said "best of luck" when Mum said she would take the 3-year-old. I said that if anything happened and she couldn't look after her then I would do so. All done! Jojo would have her teeth cleaned and a health check, we would pick her up later in the week.

The first significant thing was that I noticed spots of blood on the carpet between the bedroom and bathroom. I asked Ken about it and he was very vague. Well logic would prevail, and I would win this argument - the trail led to his side of the bed so there was little point denying there was something not right. Ken had an infuriating habit of only answering a question if he had to and only to the precise point of the inquiry. His lifetime motto was "never complain and never explain", thanks Benjamin Disraeli for encapsulating the British stiff upper lip mentality.

Eventually I was tired of cleaning the carpet each day and he admitted a problem under one of his toes. For someone who didn't complain he had no problem frequently seeking medical advice and so he went to the doctor. And again, and then again – each time with more cream to try, until finally five months later the doctor admitted that the yeast infection was a misdiagnosis.

It was one of those bizarre moments, seen in vivid contrast, when I had to choose between Ken and my mother. Ken's car was in being serviced and yet he had made another doctor's appointment. Trying to satisfy both parties I had Ken drop Mum and I off at the local mall to do some shopping. The plan was to meet back in the supermarket carpark. As we got in the car Ken pulled me aside and told me he had melanoma and he needed to go into Wellington to the specialist with some urgency, i.e., the next morning. We'll have that bombshell news with a side of Pak'n'Save shopping thanks.

* * *

The second was the dawning realisation that something was wrong with Mum was six months earlier when she failed her driving test at age 75. After some tests we were told she had the beginning stages of dementia. This was her greatest fear and had been talked about for years. Her mother also had dementia and Mum had been devastated that she needed to go into assisted care after my grandfather passed.

I didn't want to add to the lineage! I didn't want to follow in my father's footsteps and be a "stroke at 60" victim either. Talk about between a rock and a hard place when considering a healthy older age based on my parents and grandparents experiences.

Since I had been cleaning up my diet I had become "that" zealot for how everyone else could also benefit. Particularly my mother who

I could see myself in so clearly. It started with the dairy and rosacea connection. I explained it constantly but giving up cheese, butter or yoghurt wasn't going to happen. More serious though was the gluten and brain fog connection that I observed in myself and suspected was happening with her too.

Back in Christchurch in the early 2000s I would have to close the door and have a 20-minute nap if I had eaten a bread roll for lunch. Since ditching gluten, I didn't get that brain fog.

Looking at the food Mum purchased I could see an awful lot of bread products. It is often the case that people living alone and getting older will gravitate to the easy meal options, and sadly toast seems to feature prominently. I did some research online and found a few connections between diet and vascular dementia. I explained, cajoled, and offered to do the shopping. I regularly delivered dairy-free smoothies and gluten-free baking. I didn't win the battle though as they were left untouched. When she was happy to be prescribed a dairy-based supplement by her doctor it was time to admit defeat. Mum already knew that dairy was the cause of lifelong rosacea flares and I had to acknowledge in the end that it was her choice.

Traveling through Asia and interacting with my local distributor network I had experienced firsthand a number of families living with elderly parents. This really resonated with me and I had spoken to Ken about the possibility. He wasn't keen but respected that it was important to me. Now I was being placed in a position where just as I was recognising the disfunction of the Mother Daughter relationship there was a pull to go further down the "rabbit-hole".

And in the meantime Jojo was creating havoc in what had been a calm home environment. She was stealing food and getting rounder by the day. Walking her on the lead was near impossible as she was capable of pulling Mum over. I was getting regular calls to go and find her as she alternated between running away and being locked in the wardrobes. Eventually I found a compromise and they both came to stay each weekend. There was nothing idyllic about this scenario and my stress levels rocketed off the charts yet again.

CHAPTER 13

Napier 2014 - IronMāori Quarter Ironman (take 2)

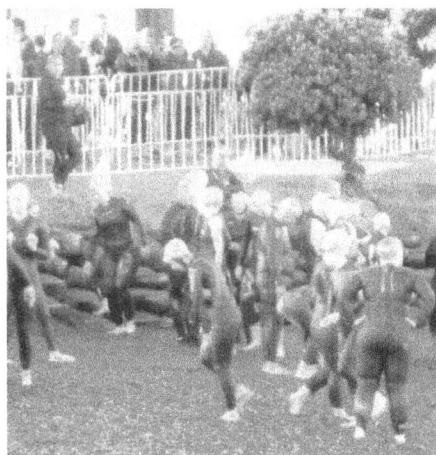

Our group was buzzing with the successes of the 2013/14 season, and we were keen to do it all again. The territory was familiar as we had trained through winter once already. The kit purchases continued as investments were made in new bikes, wind and rain-proof clothing, wind trainers and tech gadgets.

I started to read every book I could download about endurance sport and nutrition. A couple of years earlier I had succumbed and purchased a Kindle - mostly because I had been doing lots of long-distance travel and the ability to not carry books around physically was appealing.

For many years I had implemented a strategy of buying a book at the airport – proceed to read it for hours on end – and then leave it in the seat pocket of the plane or in the airport for the next person. I'm not sure I was ever on the receiving end of the "pay it forward" with books but I left many books in random places, and I love the mini lending libraries that have now popped up in our local communities.

* * *

The Kindle worked in a different fashion now. Basically, I could easily access all the books about endurance sports (particularly triathlon and ironman), nutrition and training. Following on from what I had learnt at the YTT about the importance of food, it was clear food and physical fitness were key ingredients to performance.

As I kept reading the biographies of these successful athletes it was apparent that it was not just physical fitness that was important - mental strength was the deciding factor in all the stories.

Here are a few of the key books I devoured:

- Eat and Run. Scott Jurek
- Finding Ultra. Rich Roll
- A life without limits. Chrissie Wellington
- Running with the Mind of Meditation. Sakyong Miplan
- Hot Flashes and Half Ironmans. Pamela Fagan Hutchins
- IronFit Strength Training and Nutrition. Don Fink, Melanie Fink
- Running to Extremes. Lisa Tamati

• Swim, Bike, Run, Our Triathlon Story. Alister Brownlee, Jonathon Brownlee

Some of the triathlon group were engaging coaches for their event training. I didn't feel that it was necessary at this point – preferring to do the research myself (as you can see from the reading list). I had by now invested in a Garmin GPS multisport watch and randomly signed up for their training plans. Not just one – but a few – I wanted to see what was consistent about the various programs. As a woman in my fifties, it was a very different performance story to my younger, fitter counterparts. Also, it would have been foolish to miss the opportunity to understand the cross-over between endurance training and the physical practice of yoga.

At first glance it appeared to be the stretching component that was most helpful. After a few months though, it became obvious that "core strength" is the point where yoga and training intersected. At the end of the run when you are too tired to hold yourself upright, core strength will make all the difference. I write those words with all the innocence of someone who did not know what was coming in her future.

The other factor was the ability to breathe properly. There are two points of difference between "fitness trained" and "yoga trained" when it comes to breath. The first is the ability to maintain a slow even breath for longer - important because in the moment when breath becomes shorter, this is the point when the brain signals stress and the heart rate starts to rise. The brain will call time on exertion before the body is truly done. The second is the ability to control the breath sufficiently to slow it, i.e., bio-hack the nervous system and bring the heart-rate down. Both factors result in delaying the message of fatigue, allowing the race to continue.

* * *

I would like to say I had a love-hate relationship with the gym. The reality however was I just didn't have one. As part of the registration for KWT there was a reduced membership with one of the sponsors - City Fitness. That first year I made it inside the doors and onto the treadmill on a few occasions. Mostly when it was raining outside. My big progression was to the rowing machine a couple of metres away – for a warm-up prior to the running machine. The reality was I was scared of the gym and always had been!

Back in Sydney in the mid-2000s I had joined the gym that was next door to the office on George Street in the CDB. I went in and had the personal assessment and was given a quick tour of the facilities and a personal training plan. I ventured into their yoga studio once, looked around, got freaked out by the people looking back at me and left. I got on the treadmill and pushed a few buttons and there you go – that was my gym experience sorted. Attached to the gym was a skin treatment centre. Once I had appointments in there, I used the gym as a thoroughfare to relaxing facials and treatment for that Rosacea.

This had to change now – and I engaged a personal trainer. One who had been involved with training others for the KWT. We immediately hit it off, perhaps too well as most sessions were a chat-fest as we righted the world's wrongs. I enjoyed our fitness sessions and blindly followed the instructions on what to do. I had no idea of what to do with the machines on my own. I like to push myself, and it was obvious even though I had no coordination, or natural aptitude, that what I had in spades was determination and perseverance.

What I hadn't consciously recognised to this point was how much I feared EVERYTHING. Each time it was a new exercise I hesitated. Was it just a desire to stay in a comfort zone? Or was it something much more? The dialogue in my head finally came out as I was coaxed to voice what I was thinking. I hadn't realised that I viewed everything as the potential for disaster – particularly for personal injury to myself and others. I would have made a good Health and Safety Officer. I could see the opportunity for calamity everywhere, and in effect I was living my whole life under that level of fear.

The strategy for this Quarter Ironman was for it to be a long training event to prepare me for the Half Ironman in Taupō in five weeks' time. In the comfort of shared coffee after our weekly group training sessions, it had been easy to theorise that "double the distance" was next goal.

The relief at not trying to achieve a good time in Napier was amazing. It was a time to practice the transitions and fuelling strategy. I knew that no matter how hard it was I only had to run and smile when passing the cameras.

What should have been an easy event got off to a rocky start when I tried to put my head down and swim. In the cold I just couldn't breathe. Eventually I concluded that the only way to make progress was to turn on my back and do backstroke. This was much to the horror of those around me, because then I could and did pass swimmers. I swam over a few too. There is a lesson in doing your own thing and not apologising for your actions. Our coach used to laugh in the training as all us were saying sorry all the time. She knew with event experience that politeness would get knocked out of us.

Despite the "take your time" attitude I finished third in my age group and slightly faster than the previous year. Going out slow definitely works for me in endurance events. It keeps the heart rate down and allows me to warm up fully.

* * *

Safety is a relative thing. We are inherently exposed to risk as part of being alive. Some countries you feel safe in, some parts of the country you may feel safe in. Sometimes you don't even feel safe in your one home. The worst is when you don't feel safe in your own skin.

The "love the skin you are in" is a great marketing campaign. But what if you are so disconnected from what is going on internally that you come to a point where you can't trust your body?

I recall a road trip Ken and I took at the millennium through Italy. Our diet consisted of eating bread, pasta, cheese, ham, mushrooms, and lots of wine. One day a rash appeared on my wrist. It disappeared a few hours later and I thought nothing more of it. The next day I had a similar rash on the other wrist as well as the ankles. As it had previously disappeared on its own - I ignored it. We drove from the port city of Genoa to a remote farmhouse outside of Sienna. This was true Tuscan countryside and although it was the middle of winter it was stunning. The farmhouse was beautifully renovated, we had plenty of food and wine, and artfully stacked firewood for an open fire. As we cosied up for a few days of solitude the rash came back. This time it was on my shins and arms too. I showed Ken and although it was a mild burning sensation it wasn't too bad. As the afternoon turned to evening the rash was getting worse. The strangest thing was that it was moving. It disappeared from one area to come up in another. And it was getting more intense. Soon it was covering my whole body and I felt like I was burning up from the inside out. That warm cosy environment of the Tuscan villa was my enemy and by now I was taking most of my clothes off and going outside in the cold to relieve the pain.

Could we get a doctor – or go to a doctor? How do you call an ambulance in Italian? By now I was panicking as it had occurred to us both that it could be going to affect organs and not just the skin. What on earth could it be? As the rash now covered my entire body including my face it was getting serious. Even Ken looked concerned.

Although we had both recently dealt with a bout of food poisoning from eating the mussels at an outdoor restaurant in Nice this was in a different category. I was having a health crisis of some unknown origin. We didn't even have the internet to check with Doctor Google!

While we dithered and debated what to do I wondered if I could sleep it off. Lying down and feeling waves of heat and pain moving throughout the body is an exercise in mind control. Eventually though I fell asleep. Ken stayed with me to make sure I was okay. Close to midnight I felt it was subsiding. We agreed to stay put and find help in the morning.

The next morning the rash was gone, and I was fine. How do you go to a foreign doctor and try to explain what had happened when there is no remaining physical evidence? Driving through the Italian countryside we stopped and looked at the cave dwellings. When it came to lunch and the baguette with ham and cheese, I was suddenly cautious. What if it was something I was eating? It would explain a lot. These were all things I ate – but not day after day. Was it a perfect storm of food combinations? I very much thought so.

At some level this was when I understood that I couldn't just eat anything and get away with it. However, as the days went by it was fine. By the time we returned to New Zealand it was just a bizarre tale of the trip to go along with the others like getting snowed in on Mount Blanc, accidently checking into a thalassotherapy (treatments using sea water) health spa in Biarritz. Imagine the shock on our faces going to dinner to find half the people in their white spa robes and healthy food and no alcohol. We politely declined and went out for something more substantial. Nowadays I would appreciate that option!

Eventually I understood that it wasn't just the overload of food that caused the tipping point in Italy. It was the result of the level of stress I was enduring. Between 1998 - 2000 I had experienced my father's passing, the partial sale of our company to an American investor, the bank foreclosing on our home (having clocked up no less than 3 mortgages to keep our business operating), and a brush with cervical cancer (thankfully caught early enough that an operation was all that was needed).

Stress is such an overused word, loaded with connotations and expectations of behaviour. If we substitute "pressure" it can be looked at with fresh eyes. Pressure comes from not being able to deal with the flow of events in one or more areas of life. Just like the laundry pile grows until it needs to be dealt with; if we don't process experiences as they occur, we will create a pressure point.

The yoga term is Samskaras, the subtle impressions of our past actions. The process of clearing these may be as simple as: filing away an awkward conversation so that it doesn't need to replay again and again, or as large as addressing the unprocessed grief of a family member passing.

The main categories of stressors/pressures are:

- Environmental (home, work, social, overuse of technology, exposure to chemicals)
- Emotional (unexpressed negative feelings)
- Postural (tension and misalignment)
- Nutritional (deficiencies, substances)
- Time (constraint, obsession, urgency)

Now I was challenged with the need to confront the accumulated stress because the fear (manifesting as anxiety) was limiting my actions. Not in a "face the fear and do it anyway" approach. It was time to use the physical practice of yoga to clear the issues relating to stress from my mind, via my body's memory.

In 2014 I had a "once or twice a week" yoga practice, choosing to attend a local studio. This was not enough to clear the accumulation of pressure of the current week – let alone chip away at the rest of my issues. My studio was lying idle, I needed to learn to roll out my mat for myself. For without connecting to the physical body (and all its retained stories) we cannot clear them.

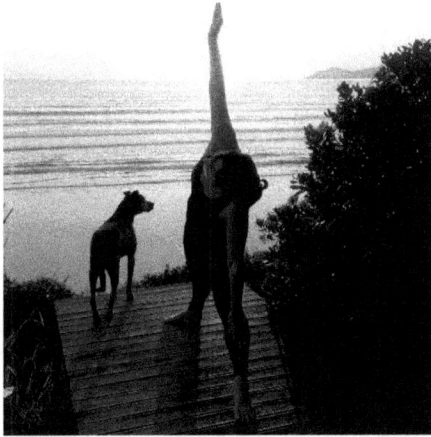

Fear keeps us small. The most noticeable manifestation of this is when we say that we can't afford to do something. More likely it is that we don't have the energy for that activity. We may have constrained ourselves in some way. A hack for this is to re-frame the statement into "this is not a priority right now". If you say that and it feels true then great, you know that it is okay to decline the opportunity. If you say it and have an immediate energetic surge, then you will make it happen.

Money is the physical representation of your energy. Understanding this allows us to change the approach – addressing the underlying cause rather than the symptoms.

The next part of this equation is when you are tired and out of money. Our mind says we need to work harder. Contrary to what we have been taught, the answer is to rest and eat well. When we re-build our energetic resources, we can be creative and manifest the funds needed.

CHAPTER 14

Wellington 2014 - Yoga Continuing Education Workshop

As part of the International Yoga Alliance membership, it is a requirement to teach for a certain number of hours each year and attend a prescribed number of hours training. I was very reluctant to return to yoga training. But was now regularly covering for a teacher at her studio – so was between a rock and a hard place. Although I had the teaching hours, I needed to get more education hours. There was a workshop in Wellington mentioned on social media. It was the right number of hours, and I didn't need to leave home. Perfect.

Ken drove me into Wellington. I was in such a fragile state I wasn't confident to take the car into the city. Once there it reinforced my negative attitude as it was everything I disliked about the yoga scene. The facilitators were wrapped up in catching up on gossip. They had no interest in the students apart from the few that belonged to their respective studios. They were being uber cool eating gluten-free cereal from the box. Trendy in the latest spiritual warrior attire. Not a good start and we hadn't even got inside the studio.

"Assisting" is an interesting concept in yoga. It allows the student to go beyond their perceived limits. Once that barrier is broken for the student then a new normal is created. The important point is that the student must be ready and willing to break through their limits and, they must not rely on the external support of the teacher to achieve the result. Otherwise, a pattern of dependency is established.

I was constantly bemoaning my lot about being back in New Zealand (and having no direction) to my mother, and her suggestion was that I become a life coach. She recognised in me the ability to see a situation for what it was and clearly communicate a way through. She knew better than anyone else - my whole life I had been giving her advice. This training module on the fundamentals of assisting clarified the concept of life coaching. It was not something I was interested in. If I was going to do anything then wanted to create something different. Why would I do what had been done before?

The quote generally attributed to Lao Tzu is "when the student is ready the teacher will appear". My negativity persisted; "Great I'm ready – where is my teacher." Within the yoga philosophy there is a history of teacher/student relationship. A direct passing down of the knowledge from the guru. A Guru is defined by Wikipedia as "mentor, guide, expert, or master".

Realistically it wasn't practical for me to up anchor and find my Guru. Life had to continue. Furthermore, I reflected on one of the eight yoga limbs – Aparigraha (non-attachment or non-possessiveness). These 8 limbs are the path to enlightenment that a yoga student follows – I like to call them the "guidebook to doing life" as they describe the ways to interact with others, society, and your physical self. The more I pondered the concept of non-attachment the more I came to believe that the notion of the guru was out of date. I believe we need to become our own guru. The knowledge is within us – we just need to find the keys to unlock it. It was at that moment the second part of the Lao Tzu quote popped up "when the student is truly ready the teacher disappears". Bingo!

When you look around, it is endemic in our society that we outsource so much. Local and central government don't maintain experts, they call in the consultants when a project needs to be undertaken. We have life coaches, health coaches, business coaches. Food can be outsourced to takeaways, ready prepared meals, food delivery services. We got so busy being busy that we forgot to look after ourselves. I believe it is more fundamental than that. It is that we no longer prioritise ourselves. Taking a 180 degree turn I also see the pattern of people helping others to the detriment of their own personal well-being. What is that story about putting the oxygen mask on – that's right – put your own on first before trying to help others.

Coming from a deep belief that the only person who will save me - is me - I stopped and double-checked whether the outside assistance was necessary. Yes, it is necessary when the person has technical skills that you don't possess. But often it is merely confirmation of that deep inner knowing. It was time to learn to trust that part within me. I was becoming my own healer and I was taking full responsibility for the state of my body and mind.

I bristle at the popular comment about "soul growth", it's not the soul that needs to grow, and many ways it's not about personal growth either. Well it is, only the approach needs to switch direction. We don't need to learn more, instead we need to unlearn that which has kept us separate from the innate knowledge already within.

This switching technique has served me well. Whether it is the 180 degree turn, the flip, or the about-turn. From this point on I approached all situations with the question of what the other side looked like. The moment I was able to move aside and consider the alternate angle I could access the Observer within. From this perspective my world looked a very different place.

CHAPTER 15

Taupō 2014 - Half Ironman

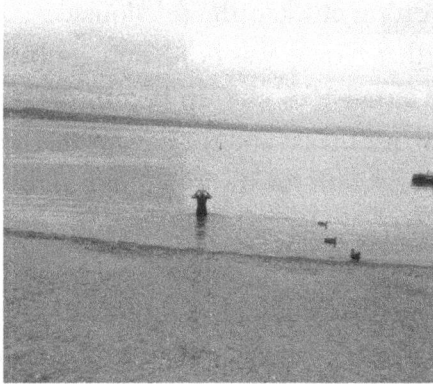

The theory is that your time for a Half Ironman will be double the Quarter distance plus an extra hour. The swim is 1.8kms, bike leg is 90kms and the run 21.2kms. At around three and a quarter hours for the three equivalent quarter events I had done in the past 18 months, it meant I was going to be out on the circuit for seven and half hours. Basically, it's the working day without lunch and tea breaks. This is about twice the time that the elite athletes take. It means that those of us towards the back will still be on the course during the hottest part of the day. Like a half marathon that you may be able to wing through, but not the marathon; the books were saying you can't "wing your way through a Half Ironman. It needs to be taken seriously and prepared for.

This was the motivation I was looking for to break through the impasse I was in. I would approach it as seriously as I had done for my first Quarter Ironman. Even better I would invite some of my training buddies to join me.

As part of the preparation for the event I stopped eating all meat. I gave up red meat eight years earlier as I found it always made me incredibly tired the next day. Now the experts say it can take up to two days to fully digest. Those books I was reading had a theme of improved performance centred on a plant-based diet. I noticed that my legs felt heavy because of eating chicken the previous day. There was another unaddressed food that I knew was not helping – bacon. It's interesting how many people struggle to give up bacon, me included. Really it's not about the meat, it's the fat and the flavour that we get addicted to. I started playing around with substituting smoked fish in the recipes and it worked well for me.

With the benefit of hindsight, I believe that a key part of my overcoming the fear that permeated my life was giving up meat. Meat carries the energetic vibration of the fear that the animal experiences at death. We imbibe that and it becomes part of our energetic shape too. Fear is a basic human instinct; it comes from a stress response of some description, external (the proverbial tiger) or internal (inflammation, excess adrenalin). I had enough of it already and didn't need more.

I was living in a body that was becoming strong and my confidence was growing. The best strategy for me was breaking the event down into bite size pieces. If I didn't think beyond the current activity, I was able to stay in a positive mindset of it being "doable".

In the past two years I had done more than I thought was even physically possible. This event was never going to be about the time. It was a challenge about who I was becoming. I knew many areas where I could do better, but I had a clear realisation that there would be another set of circumstances to be dealing with next time. It was becoming okay to be "good enough".

Even though it was my first half Ironman I felt relaxed and ready. I knew the course, and like the Taupō environment. There is something very special about swimming in the lake. Maybe it's the lack of waves and fresh water, personally I think there is a special spirit within the lake.

It was Ken's birthday a few days earlier. We took time to visit Rotorua and then he dropped me in Taupō to meet the others.

The swim once again was a mass start – I was prepared to seed myself closer to others. We floated and waited for the starter's gun. I remembered the Coach's advice about having a pee (yes in the wetsuit in the water) before I got started. I wondered if that was what everyone was doing. Best not to think too much when you are about to put your head down and start breathing through that water. The long bike ride out to Reporoa requires discipline as it is a mental game as well as physical. There is a significant uphill gradient in the last 15kms back into Taupō that needs to be factored in. Coming out of the swim well is a great feeling but then seeing everyone pass you is soul-destroying. I needed a reminder that this was my competition with myself. Time to focus on the van that was tailing the last cyclists – picking up those that would not make the cut-off. All I needed to do was to be back in transition before the van.

There was relief to eventually be on the run course - now I was in control of my destiny. I had the healthy snacks and plenty of drinks. I had a "better than a ringside" ticket to watch the elite athletes finishing their day. Although I was completing the event for the first time (and for myself), there was no sense of pride or accomplishment. It was just done.

* * *

Did I mention "menopause"? By now I was 53 and fully in the grip of the "change". Over 20 years on the contraceptive pill had significantly impacted my hormones.

Going on the pill was not something I questioned. My career was important, and (since I was a teenager) I thought I didn't want children. Growing up in the 70's it was the obvious answer to birth-control. I just didn't get the memo that said I should stop at some point. Even after the cancer scare – the surgeon had said that I could still have children (now aged 39). No issue, in fact Ken thought I could have a hysterectomy as part of the operation. That was a line I wouldn't cross; he wouldn't have a vasectomy. Solution I would continue to take the pill. All decided without consideration for the consequences on my body.

No surprise a year later when I did an about turn and decided I did want to have a child after all. And then started a litany of miscarriages from ages 41 – 46. The first being the most memorable as we were in San Francisco and presenting to a multi-national telecommunications giant. The last being on the train home from the Sydney CBD on Christmas Eve.

Reading about menopause symptoms I came across articles that suggested not having children was a contributing factor to the severity of the symptoms. Well, I fitted that profile, plus some. What had started three years earlier as an unwelcome 50th birthday gift, an uncontrollable nuisance, was now something I had to learn to manage holistically.

I quickly learnt that I could not "look" at spicy food without breaking into a sweat. Making for interesting family dinners as I mopped sweat from my entire body. Especially unpleasant if I had been swimming in the pool earlier. At that point I instigated a regimen of spending time in the sauna after swim training. This practice effectively cleared the chlorine from the pores of my skin, and I'm sure resulted in less chemical absorption, further helping my ongoing detoxification process.

One question that came up was regarding eating tofu and soy milk. It really helped reduce the severity of my hot flushes. So much so I started purchasing blocks of soft tofu and using that in smoothies instead of almond milk. Win-win as I have a pet hate for those Tetra Pak cartons that alternative milks are packaged in, as they are not recyclable. For me it was becoming important to look at the bigger picture - factoring in the effect on the environment as well as its impact on my physical self.

It was easy to ditch the caffeine and alcohol as both were not conducive to sleeping well and being refreshed for training five days a week. In order to fit in 2-3 swims, 1 long bike ride, and 3 run sessions a week it became necessary to double up some days. And as the run distances got longer it was sometimes an option to run twice in one day. No surprise when I look back and say that "weight-gain during menopause" was something that bypassed me. Best to take the small wins when they present themselves.

* * *

I wondered how much of the aching muscles and legs, sore joints and exhaustion was the training, and how much was related to hormonal changes occurring. It was time to add an understanding of the body's hormone system to the equation.

My first step towards balancing my hormone system was to turn to food as medicine. By now I was very familiar with macro nutrients (carbohydrates, protein and fats) but less so with the impact of micro nutrients in the form of vitamins and minerals. Randomly I would pop a multi-vitamin daily for a few weeks until I forgot. Always thinking that I was probably just creating expensive urine.

The body has a fantastic feedback system - if only I would notice - and now I was aware that as I was getting depleted I would start to get mouth ulcers. I increased my Vitamin C with a small glass of lemon water each day. Ditching chocolate wasn't happening but amazing handmade raw chocolate bars were becoming popular in the health stores and I probably singlehandedly kept at least one brand in business. Raw cacao is high in antioxidants, iron and magnesium - all helping me with those micro nutrients on a daily basis.

CHAPTER 16

Byron Bay 2015 - YTT

I still hadn't solved the yoga pants issue. I had my running gear. Seriously, I had a lot of running gear. I had no problem with signing into Wiggle UK and buying all the gear I needed for a triathlon. I had long pants, knee length pants, shorts, sports bras. I was sure enough of myself to even buy the BlueSeventy wetsuit online. But I did not own a pair of yoga pants. I was wearing my training gear for yoga which just made me hot and uncomfortable. And now most of those were compression pants. Not at all suitable for belly breathing. On the last day of the course the studio had a pop-up store. This was still a step too far – but one that needed to be taken. All the styles and sizes were in front of me. Why couldn't I just buy a pair and be done with it. It was too much. I walked away.

Recall those supportive women on yoga retreats? They saw that I didn't follow through on the yoga pants issue and physically took my hand and stood by until I bought the first pair – now I need to be reminded to wear proper clothes.

As part of the retreat package there were two sports massages included. Those that had been to Byron Bay trainings before were excited. I was apprehensive.

My first massage was at the age of 40. My mother gave me a gift voucher for my birthday. I'm sure she saw the look of disgust on my face at that present. And worse was the need to redeem it before I left the Hawkes Bay a few days later. To her credit she had not actually booked the appointment. I had to make the phone call myself. Now that was going outside my comfort zone. Go to a strange house, take most of your clothes off, lie on a bed and relax. You have got to be kidding me. I lay rigid until the last minute or so, at that point my whole body jerked and I just about kicked myself off the bed. That is a good definition of wired.

At the appointed time I headed over in my running gear for the massage. I am chronically early to everything. Which only adds to the anticipation/fear as I invariably must wait. As he started sticking his elbows into my muscles, my internal dialogue was "Relax, relax, breathe deeply, this is good for you." As we concluded he mentioned that I had a high pain tolerance. No kidding. He had only ever seen one other case like me. A high-flying executive from Sydney who could and did tolerate pain to that level without flinching. Little did he know that my background was exactly that. I laughed it off and we put it down to all the endurance training I was doing.

The experience was cause for reflection – When was I not in pain? When didn't I have a headache? Never and never. I may trick myself that I didn't need medication, but I was also deluding myself about the state I was in.

There are so many types of headache: tension, stress, migraine. They all have a negative impact on your wellbeing. I mean, how is it possible to be happy when your head is thumping. Or your eye feels like it will explode. As I became healthier my headaches reduced but if I eat processed foods, then next day I can physically see the puffiness down the left side of my face. Some processed foods are easy to identify; we know them by their brand name rather than a food group. More recently is the trend towards new manufactured products that are perceived as good for us and the planet. My simplest guide – if it has a 3-digit code as an ingredient – I, and my body, do not recognise it as food.

Another pain quote is from Rumi – I even put it in the forward of the recipe book. "Listen to these pains they are messengers". With the benefit of hindsight regarding my own journey, as well as dozens of clients showing up with matching physical and emotional symptoms, it's not hard to see recurring patterns as to where we hold certain life experiences.

I never did see the twin towers come down in 2001. Firstly, I didn't own a TV set at the time and secondly, I was flying that morning from Christchurch to Wellington for a business meeting with a government department. I went to get out of bed and my shoulder seized up. Welcome to my first "frozen shoulder" experience. A couple of Panadol and I was on my way to the airport – trying to carry a heavy bag. Trying to prepare for the meeting. Trying to smile and be friendly, relaxed, and personable. All in incredible agony.

Did I have the weight of the world on my shoulders at that time? Yes, the company wasn't doing well and we had been forced to sell our house 18 months earlier. Days earlier I had returned from the US, during which time we were negotiating to buy a US manufacturer. It was my 40th birthday while we were away. My grandmother had passed away and I hadn't made it back in time for the funeral. Ken was still in the US to conclude the negotiations.

* * *

This YTT was about "Hanuman" the Hindu God that took the form of a monkey. He was unaware of his true powers and while helping his masters in one of their ordeals he needed to take a "leap of faith", overcome his doubts and access his latent potential.

Doubt is a feeling rather than an emotion. It is coming from the mind. If it is self-doubt it stems from a lack of confidence. The good news is that feelings can always be re-framed. Catch them early enough and they can be turned to the affirmative.

Fresh with enthusiasm from the YTT, I started to explore the idea of "fasting". I was well into fresh juices and using food to heal. Various internet searches kept bringing me back to this. The concept of voluntarily going without food for a period of time was incomprehensible to me. Maybe it was time to bust through that limit as well. I am the person that does things in very small slow steps. Not the jump in "boots'n'all" personality. Each month around the full moon I embarked on a period of only consuming liquids – smoothies, juices and soups. Sometimes I would make 24 hours, other times I was able to push it out to around 60 hours. Most of my internal doubt and dialogue was amplified by the people around me. Eventually it was better not to say what I was doing.

CHAPTER 17

Dubai 2015 - Yoga Immersion Course

I needed to go back to Dubai to wrap up the last of the business activities. I was understandably very reluctant – until the opportunity came to immerse myself in some more yoga training. Only then was I prepared to weigh up the trauma of going through immigration, and deem it worthwhile, to get back into the United Arab Emirates.

After three years of eating healthily in New Zealand it was a shock to be buying and consuming food in Dubai. Initially it looked like an amazing array of fresh fruit and vegetables. Until you read the packaging – almost everything was air-freighted in from overseas. The main locally grown produce are tomatoes and cucumbers. And the best fresh dates in the world. Talking to my yoga colleagues everyone was taking vitamin supplements of some description. Apparently, there was not enough nutrients in the food. There was a great appreciation for how lucky we are in New Zealand to have a climate that supports an abundance of fresh food. "Local and in-season" is my criteria to avoid needing extra vitamins. Partly because I resent pee-ing out dollars, mainly because vitamins are not going to raise the energetic vibration of the body.

At the same time I began an almost "vigilante" attack on all things chemical in my life. This included the products I was using on my body as well as those around the home. Ken had the same approach to insects, having no trouble emptying half an aerosol can in the pursuit of a single fly. I unplugged the air fresheners and insect repellents and began burning incense. A bit like the question of when is it too soon to start the vacuum cleaner after family have visited for the holidays – when to light the sage to clear the environment of any negative energy? Answer - it is never too soon - just do it.

I noticed an interesting phenomenon – less meat in my diet equalled less body odour. As I slowly removed the chemicals there was a distinctly metallic odour for a while. And then nothing at all!

There is something surreal about catching a taxi into the ultra modern and sterile financial district of Dubai, walk into the air-conditioned yoga studio and spending the day moving and learning. A couple of the women from the initial training were there. We spent the week discussing the yoga philosophy as it relates to modern life.

Alongside the yoga, were trips to the bank, the trade office, and my clients. Everything fell into place to such an extent that the clients from Riyadh were in town for a few days and keen to catch up. It had been three years now since I had actively been working the business. I was absolutely delighted to see clients - some of whom I had known for over ten years. What was now impossible for me was the concept of a "sales pitch". There were opportunities presented – and in the past I would have been the first to explore what could be done. But not now!

I was fit – fit enough for back-to-back ride classes at the fitness studio. Sitting on the bike staring at the full-length mirrors at the front of the class I noticed my left shoulder was about 20 centimetres higher than the right. I thought "that's a bit weird" as I tried to pull it down.

It was my first moment of clarity as to how tension shows up as actual physical misalignment in the body. This was the result of that frozen shoulder some years earlier.

When the knees are causing problems the first question to ask is where you are holding back in moving forward with life. Louise Hay's book "You can Heal yourself" is the seminal work regarding body and emotional connections. Hip issues have a lot to do with feeling safe and secure in the world. Often hip issues stem from knee issues that haven't been dealt with.

It took me a long time to see the correlation, and then more time to realise that we can positively impact ourselves to clear these patterns. Not just learn how to cope with something, but truly let the trauma go. It takes effort to do work on yourself. We can go to the chiropractor, acupuncturist, massage therapist, reiki healer; and they will give short-term relief that will provide a glimpse as to how things could be. But eventually, as part of the journey of personal growth, it is necessary to do the clearing work ourselves.

Why don't we help ourselves? The ego/mind has a vested interest in keeping things the way they are. The mind votes for the status quo. The body and higher self vote together for the greater good. It's why we don't do what we know is good for us. For example, how often do the healthy foods stay at the back of the pantry?

Spending a week on the yoga mat with an internationally renowned US yoga teacher was confronting! This was my check-in as to where I truly was. All those pains, tensions and physical limitations can be seen and felt, I needed strength and courage to work through them. I was ready to take that leap.

As I boarded the plane to return to New Zealand my journal entry read:

"Responsibility vs Obligation". These are not the same thing! I have a responsibility to myself and Buster (as he is dependent on me) but not to anything else. I have obligations as a wife, daughter, and sister. But let me remind myself that these are not my responsibilities."

It has been three years since I left Dubai under a black cloud. Ignoring it has not made it go away. So this time some light has been shed on the situation and I finally understand the lesson. The fear is real – but not for the situation. That was in the past and I survived it. What I did not do is recognise it for what it was. Now I do. So now I'm ready, I will book my return flight – get on the plane – fly back to New Zealand – and move on with my life.

These last three weeks have been about re-connecting with the yoga path. Not just the physical practice – all 8 limbs."

CHAPTER 18

Taupō 2015 - Marathon

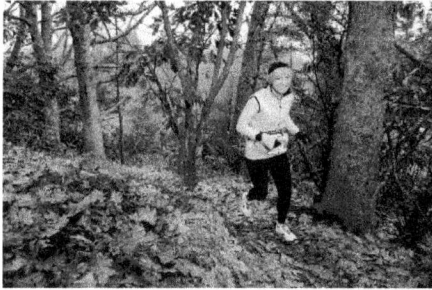

Each of my events fell apart at the run stage. I didn't have the physical endurance or the mental fortitude to continue to run. In fact, apart from my first endurance event, I hadn't completed a triathlon without walking most of the run leg. I recognised this at the Wellington Half Marathon a few months earlier and had decided to do something about it.

Now situations were popping up to help me deal with this limitation. And they were all culminating in the decision to run my first full marathon. All 42.2kms of it. But I didn't just choose a flat road course. No, I was doing the inaugural Taupō marathon which was half trail and half road, and it was in the middle of winter at altitude. This meant freezing temperatures and snow and ice were a possibility.

First it came from a seed planted by my Personal Trainer and I had the opportunity to connect with an endurance running group. They were interested in the 35 Day Detox for their online group. I was interested in learning more about how to run long-distance. I embraced this new direction and headed away for a run-training weekend for women. Running on the trails of Lake Mangamahoe in Taranaki was incredible.

I was born and raised in New Plymouth and to be back in the Taranaki bush was good for my soul. Gone was the young girl in the small town (population 32,387 in 1961) who couldn't run or do sport. The one who as a teenager was too timid to do tumble turns in the pool, so she gave up competitive swimming, and turned to surf-lifesaving instead. Then when the movie Jaws was released, freaked out about being in the open water too.

Secondly, I was riding high on the success of facing my fear of returning to Dubai. Running the Dubai Marina circuit was an opportunity to see how far I had come, both in terms of physical fitness, and mental strength.

However what had started as another girl's weekend away to Taupō quickly crumbled as everyone had other priorities. I still had the house booked but there was only one other couple coming (and they had accommodation elsewhere). I suggested to Ken that he come and join me.

Leading up to the event was traumatic (and it would have made a lot of sense to have withdrawn from the event), but I don't quit easily, and this was testing my mental strength. My mother was finding it harder to live on her own and now spent each weekend at our place. Ken was looking for a new interest. I was focussing on the endurance events and the 35 Day Detox recipe book. After much discussion we decided to sell in Kāpiti and look at a vineyard in the Wairarapa. Somewhere I could hold yoga retreats. /and a place where Mum and Jojo could live with us fulltime. We put the house on the market – the first open home was August 1ˢᵗ and the day before we drove to Taupō for the Marathon. The plan was to drop Buster at the "doggie retreat" outside Shannon. Ken would be my support. I had done the training and was excited to have the chance to run through the Taupō thermal area, and then be back on familiar territory for the latter part of the race. It was the same as the Taupō Half Ironman, a course that took us out to 5-mile Bay and returned along the lakefront.

As we drove up the kennels' drive there was a lot of dogs barking. We pulled up and met the owner. Buster did not want to get out of the car, which was unlike him. We saw the accommodation – which were basic huts in a fenced area. Not "inside" as described on the website. They had gone so far as to call it a retreat rather than the standard kennels. I thought we had the wrong place. This was the middle of winter. I made a flippant comment about Buster barking as we left, and how it would be hard to bear. The owner's answer was that she just turned the hose on barking dogs – it apparently shut them up right away.

We did drive away with me shaking like a leaf. I couldn't believe we were leaving a well-loved old dog in such a place. The only conversation in the car was about "did we do the right thing". I called my friend who is a bit of a dog whisperer to check if she could get a sense of if he was going to be alright. She called back to say Buster was frightened and didn't know why we had left him there, but that he would be fine. Clearly that was not a good enough answer. An hour later at Bulls I was still questioning what we had done. Ken said "make a decision now." We went back and picked Buster up, gave the money to the woman, and got out as quickly as we could.

That left us with a problem of a dog going to a book-a-bach that had a no-dog policy. I started to scroll my phone in a panic for places in Taupō that we could drop Buster off at. Eventually Ken told me to "stop looking" and "we would just leave him in the car for the night". And "he would sort it the next morning". Eight hours later we arrived in Taupō (usually a four plus hour drive) and settled ourselves in. Of course, Buster came inside and I was freaking out that the neighbours would call the owners. So much for a calm lead up to my first marathon.

The following morning we went for a drive to see where the race started and took Buster for a walk in the bush. Calming down, we decided to have brunch in town and then return to the house and make some calls to sort out Buster's accommodation. Registration was opening in the afternoon at 3pm. I had planned to have a 20-minute power nap and save my legs for the next day.

The only call I made that afternoon was "111". Ken developed a massive headache, then started to have pains and spasms in his left side. Initially we thought it was dehydration from the previous day's extended drive. When it didn't subside, it was time to call an ambulance. As the medics stabilised him, they wanted to take him to Taupō hospital for some tests. He insisted I didn't join him. Instead I was to go and register – his reasoning being that if he was okay in an hour or two, I would kick myself for not having registered.

After registration I drove to the hospital to find Ken charming the nurses. We waited for the results. Buster was still in the car – no we hadn't sorted that situation out! Eventually the decision was made that Ken needed to go to the bigger hospital in Rotorua. They wanted him in overnight to monitor him in case he had another seizure. He was adamant that I wasn't to go with him. And that I should run the next morning. So much so he had prepped the Doctor and nurses. He was proud of me and what I was doing, and I knew it.

I went back to the house and called my coaches to discuss whether to run or not. They wonderfully said if I didn't, they would run with me at a later time so that I could still "do a marathon". I decided not to decide. Rather to try and get some sleep and make a call in the morning. It was close to midnight and my alarm was set for 5am.

The next next morning my perverse reasoning when I hadn't had a call from the hospital overnight was there was nothing I could do – at least it wasn't bad news - and once they called to let me know he was being discharged I would pick him up – an hour's drive away. By now I was functioning on adrenaline and IT would just get done. Whatever "it" was - there was no room for debate as to the reasonableness of my actions.

The decision was to run. What to do with Buster? He was okay to wait in the car as he was less nervous in the car than anywhere else. But he needed a run before settling down to sleep for the morning. That meant running with him for a couple of kilometres before meeting my friend to get on the bus out to the start line. I decided to leave my phone on in case the hospital called.

Time to do my first marathon. It was as beautiful as I imagined, the approach was to run with my friend to start with, then we would go our separate ways. I kept slowing my pace to check where she was. Unfortunately, she was struggling, she had come into the race after having been sick with a chest infection for a couple of weeks. All credit to her that she stuck it out and finished the event. In hindsight I think the slow start was what saved the day for me. After about 7kms I decided that I would just do my own thing, sticking to a target pace for each 10kms of the course, the final 2.2kms target was "to keep running no matter what".

Eating and drinking consistently early in the race was a key part of my plan. I had done lots of research and been testing various foods in previous events. I had fresh dates and homemade energy balls with cacao nibs. These were rationed to 2 balls every 5kms. I had even purchased a hi-vis jacket with multiple pockets to accommodate the food. I interspersed water with a juice combination of coconut water, lemon, honey and salt. Dates are used in the Middle East to break the fast at Ramadan. They are high in natural sugar as well as having minerals such as Iron, Potassium, Copper and Magnesium. They are one of the few dried fruits that do not have any chemical additives and are ridiculously cheap for their nutritional benefits.

I continued to run until the 41km point. I was running down beside the lake and almost back into town when the phone rang. My worst nightmare, or good news? I hadn't heard from Ken at this point. My heart stopped, and so did I, to take the call. Yes I was still running after four hours. Unbelievably it was my mother calling to see how I was – I hung up on her and switched off the phone. I walked most of the last kilometre in dismay and then ran through the finish line. If I had previously doubted the connection between me stopping and my mother – I didn't ever again. Nor did I go into that dark place on a run again.

Having finished my first marathon, I headed straight for the car to get Buster and let him out for some fresh air and a pee. Celebrations, sore legs and exhaustion would have to wait. I headed back to the house for a quick shower before loading the destination "Rotorua Hospital" into the GPS and going to see what was happening with Ken.

* * *

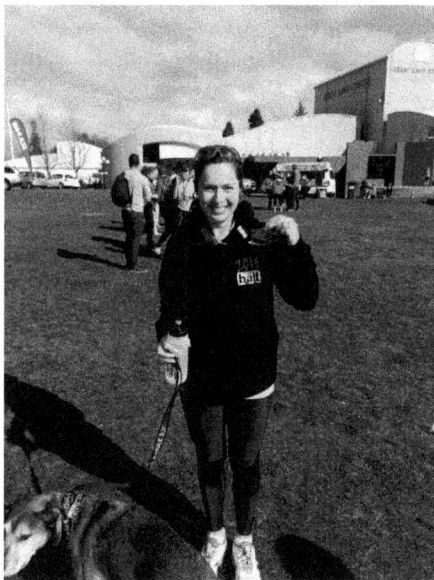

The original plan was I would have nearly week at home after Taupō before I was flying out to Bali for yet another YTT retreat. Our house was on the market and a new life was beckoning. As the hospital staff did not know what had caused the seizures we were stuck in limbo – Ken in Rotorua and me in Taupō. I was unable to move to a hotel closer as I still had Buster with me. So, it was a daily drive of 80kms each way for me. Luckily, I was able to extend my stay at the house. Perhaps not so if the owners had known I had a dog sleeping on the bed each night.

* * *

This "new life" had been crafted by taking all the pieces of the current situation and rehashing them until they came together. It was the world of compromise taken to its ultimate end-point. There was no spark of creativity, or dreams of what more is possible. I was looking to please everyone and work with the hand I had been dealt. Also I had no expectation of anything changing - other than the changes we could see within our present situation. It wasn't wrong per se, just not what the Universe had in mind for us all.

CHAPTER 19

Bali 2015 - YTT

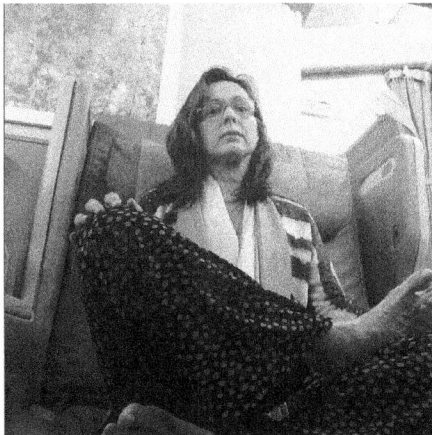

Ken was discharged from hospital, and we came back to Kāpiti, he was booked for more tests in Wellington Hospital in a couple of weeks' time.

Sensible decisions were sometimes lacking in our relationship, and he convinced me to go to Bali and I was happy to oblige.

My Auckland airport journal entry:

"8/8/8 (2+0+1+5) Infinite Possibilities.

A day for new starts. Been a while since I flew Singapore Airlines. And really Auckland airport hasn't changed in the 30 years I've been going through the terminals. Feeling very anxious waiting to board. Not sure if it's the sugar/alcohol combo, or something else. But quite upset at this point.

I love to go away – and really didn't want "nothing" to happen in my life but then it gets scary. So the reason for this trip? Primarily it is a follow-on from the yoga teaching I did in Dubai. I guess that asked more questions than it answered. And I thought it would be good to deepen the inquiry (philosophy), let's call it what it is..."

Right after the Marathon I had arranged to fly to Bali to continue my YTT. Maybe it was my ego that got me into this, or was it the wheels of fate turning once more?

One of the trainers from my original YTT posted on social media about a competition to win entry to a two-week training in Ubud, Bali. The subject was "What were you going to do differently as Yoga Teachers that would make a difference in the world?"

My submission was written that evening while sitting on the couch watching TV with Ken. I wanted to show the connection between doing yoga, and how it helps with personal development and fitness without using any of the traditional yoga Sanskrit terminology. i.e. make it accessible for all. Sacrilegious. The submission should not have even got into a serious yoga teaching shortlist. Sanskrit is an integral part of yoga as it embodies the healing sounds and vibrations that deepen the benefits of doing yoga. I might as well have said that the breath is unimportant.

Not so, a few weeks later I received an email to say I hadn't won, but I was a runner up and they were offering a 50% discount if I wanted to join the group. Great marketing strategy. The key word was "a", you guessed it – there were several of us who fronted up under that guise.

I had tried to put the yoga teaching experience of Dubai 2011 behind me. Yet I had been pulled back incessantly, and pushed out of my comfort-zone again and again. Even as the doors closed on that first training retreat in July 2011 and I thought it was over - it wasn't! It turned out that after the 150 in-person hours I would need to complete a series of three essays, plus do 20 hours of actual "teaching". Nope, that wasn't happening. I was adamant but my friend said if you have come this far why not complete it – and then at least you will have the certification. My answer "I'm not teaching so I don't need the certificate". Her answer "I have scheduled you to cover a class tonight at the gym – there will only be half a dozen people – good to cut your teeth there". After that I rocked up and did lots of cover-classes over the Dubai summer. This is the time when it is too hot to even go outside and everyone that can has left the country. I hadn't as we were preparing for the boat party. Once or twice I only had one student show up, my favourite was when nobody showed. All the stress and worry beforehand was completely wasted, but way better than the stress of actual teaching.

That is until the day I was in class at my local Dubai Marina fitness studio. I had progressed from hiding at the back of the class to now being in the front row. Well, if I had all the training then it's impossible to pretend that I had no idea what I was doing. I may have been as graceful as a hippo, but I knew what was coming next in the classes now. The teacher didn't show up; 30 people stretching, chatting, or chilling but the buzz was that we should have started by now. The receptionist came in and rather than announce anything to the class – stopped at me and asked if I would take the class. Should've stayed at the back of the class!

All mic'd up and on stage. This was a moment of truth. It was only an hour and then it would be over. I looked out and saw some of the people I had chatted with over the last few months. Namaste, "the light in me recognises the light in you". Not so for all – the only other Kiwi in the room was in the front centre two rows back. She stood up, rolled up her mat and walked out.

* * *

This 2015 YTT had a very different feel to it. The initial training four years earlier had included elements such as the sacred circle, healthy eating, and the art of living a good life. This focussed more on sequencing a class and creating a business from yoga. Both have their place, and we learn as much from what we resonate with as we do from that which we don't.

Ubud is in the central part of the island of Bali. It is a mecca for the alternative lifestyle, with green smoothies, juice bars and cafes in abundance. In contrast, extracurricular activities for this yogi group included finding a good burger and cold beer.

Ken always liked to explain the origins of the sandwich. His story comprised the Earl of Sandwich who wanted to eat meat while out on the hunt. It wasn't convenient to bring the silver cutlery with the hounds, but two slices of bread kept the aristocratic fingers clean. I had eaten my last burger in September 2011, with my family at Johnny Rockets in the Dubai Mall. I only had it to fit in with everyone and it made me so sick that to this day I have not eaten another. The combination of meat, cheese, and bread is a digestive disaster waiting to happen! Add fries and a fizzy drink and you have probably created the most indigestible meal known to mankind.

* * *

The yoga training was two one-week modules – with the options to do either or both. I wanted to do both weeks but also wanted to do the marathon. The compromise was skipping the first week and arriving in time for the second. It is never a good idea to join a group that has already been established for a week, especially in the intensely personal space of the YTT. There were a handful of people that started with me. I was one of the oldest – sharing a room with one of the youngest – an interesting combination that worked well.

There is a format to YTT retreats. Each morning starts with a 1-2 hour yoga session. Followed by time to journal/reflect – become present to the day and identify thoughts that have surfaced. Breakfast not only "breaks the overnight fast" with consumption of food, but also the first communications with others. After this is the main teaching for 2-3 hours. Mostly sitting on the floor listening. The afternoon is time for lunch and to individually (or within a group) work on the lessons of the morning. Reconvening early evening for a second yoga practice and to present to the material we have been tasked with (practice teaching, presentation, etc). Then the day is finished – well not quite – it is usual to be given homework for the next day as well. I love how that is defined as a "retreat"!

I had just finished six months of intensive training for my first marathon, run the marathon, spent a week sitting and driving 160kms a day, and sat on a plane for 10 hours. My hips were screaming blue murder. Sitting on the floor was agony. This was my healing crisis relating to the first chakra. Those issues of safety and security had their physical manifestation as chronic tightness in the hip area. It should have been a hint when I could only sleep curled up in the foetal position. Underlying that is a belief system relating to being a sovereign individual. That I had the right to be here. At least I was in the right place to get advice on the best hip stretches to start with – the answer is the humble low lunge.

Diving directly into the yoga philosophy was what I needed. Perhaps not the "what is the meaning of life" questions. But what are the factors that influence us. These are the "kleshas", roughly translated as "poisons that affect our mental state" and are the cause of suffering.

They are:

- Ignorance
- Egoism
- Attachment
- Avoidance
- Fear of Death

With the experience of "building mental strength by tackling my limiting thoughts" centre-stage, it was a great time to explore "WHY" I did certain things. I was fresh from conquering the narcissism but hadn't considered my role in the dynamic. I could lay blame for the first 18 years but why hadn't I taken responsibility for my actions as I became an adult? The issue of co-dependency jumped right out and hit me between the eyes.

Equally interesting was the concept that we change completely at age 54. The closest I could get to an astrological reason was the Saturn Return. These take place in everyone's life as the planet Saturn crosses the place it was in the skies when you were born. It is associated with major life cycles at ages 28-30 and 56-58. For me Saturn sits in Capricorn (24 degrees 42 minutes), my sixth house (daily routines, including work, health and wellness), and Capricorn's influence would manifest as a need for structure in those daily routines as well as care for myself.

The only response the young male yoga teacher could give was that his father had morphed into something very different in that year. Interesting because in two days' time I was turning 54. The logical fact-based person in me needed something more to convince me that life was being tossed in the air as we spoke.

On my birthday I spoke to Ken from Bali and he assured me that everything was fine. The drugs were keeping him stable and he didn't have any test results. Strangely he didn't call again for the next few days. Over the years we had always spoken every day no matter which of us was traveling - I was caught up in the deep dive into yoga and was grateful for the space he was giving me.

The night of my birthday – we did what all good yogis do at night to celebrate the end of the day. You guessed it – chant. Since I wasn't compelled to give the solo rendition of Sri Ram Jai Jai Ram it was strangely comforting when they chose that song as my birthday tribute. Later we went across the road to the local hotel for a glass of wine.

When I arrived back at Wellington airport Ken was there to meet me. He looked fine and said everything was great. And then as we stood at the baggage carousel, he couldn't hold the pretence any longer. "I've got 3-12 months left: the cancer has moved into my brain. Oh there's your bag." I was stunned. People were jostling for their bags all around me and I couldn't move.

I will always have this advice for myself and others - next time you are standing in a crowd and there are people acting weirdly – you have no idea what their back story is. Give them some kindness and compassion.

I had just turned 54 and Ken and I had been together half my life. Our first date had been on the 8/8/8 (1+9+8+8 = 26, 2+6 = 8), a coincidence I don't think so.

I recalled my first Saturn Return. It was about a year after Ken and I got together. Ken was one of the co-founders of the company and I was the Chief Financial Officer. Understandably the other two founders were concerned about the ethics of us having a personal relationship. I didn't take the subsequent changes well. We had a regular dinner date each Friday evening at the local Italian restaurant. I couldn't deal with the loss of my career. The fallout at the end of that week included me getting very drunk at the restaurant, locking myself in the bathroom and bawling my eyes out. And that was before the appetiser. I was taken home in disgrace.

I hoped that I had grown as a person now. Ken had come into my life at the first Saturn Return and he was leaving at the second. It wasn't just a chapter in my life ending, it felt more like it was the entire set of the Encyclopaedia Britannica had been thrown down.

CHAPTER 20

Blenheim 2016 - 100km Forrest Graperide

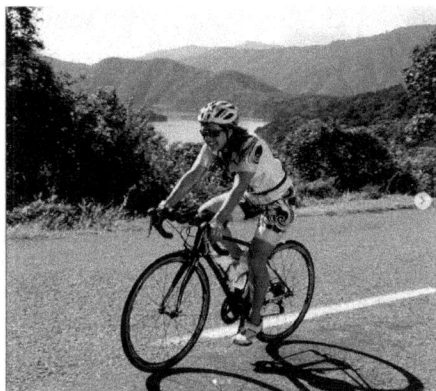

My long-distance triathlon foray seemed to have come to a natural conclusion. I was dealing with Ken's illness and trying to keep my own wellbeing in check. There was a thin strand of connection remaining to the training group in the form of a weekly group bike ride. Finally, I was beginning to enjoy being on the bike, including the downhills. The suggestion was to finish the summer season off with the Blenheim based 100km Forrest Graperide event. This event started and finished at the

Forrest Estate Winery. The course goes in a large loop from Blenheim to Picton, over the scenic Queen Charlotte Drive to Havelock, with half a dozen hills and a maximum elevation of 200m. Definitely a need for climbing legs. Good thing in my new guise as an endurance athlete I had taken to watching the Tour-de-France on Sky TV. For the female event virgins there was the chance at the end of the race to jump into the barrel and follow the tradition of stomping the grapes with your feet. I hope they tossed those grapes in the compost after we left town.

* * *

It was a surreal weekend away. I had mixed feelings about leaving Ken behind, but I really needed some time out to get a perspective on what was happening. One thing I've noticed over the years is that it's hard to get clarity on a situation when you are in it. Having some physical distance and looking back into it is a way to rise above the day-to-day stuff you are dealing with and see what is important. From that view-point you can see what can be dropped, and what can be done to change the position you find yourself in.

Catching an early morning ferry across the Cook Strait from Wellington to Picton is always an uplifting experience. Even when the weather is less than ideal. The raw elemental nature of the journey cleanses and transforms. There is the safe harbour of Wellington, and then the narrow exit past Barrett Reef and Steeple Rock Lighthouse into the open water. The crossing itself has the feeling of the unknown and potential danger. And ultimately, entry into Marlborough Sounds with its dramatic scenery of towering bush covered hills. This final cruise of an hour builds with anticipation for the sight of the port of Picton, the gateway at the top of the South Island, and the new adventure about to unfold.

The trip across the two islands connects us to our life force, to the essence of who we are. Call it prana, chi, mana. We build it by being in nature, breathing, or from others. Water is life, wind heralds change, and the hills evoke the dragon-energy.

Once again there was the comradery of a shared goal and time away to connect at a deeper level. A couple of us chose the easy option for the event – one that included a coffee stop. Sounds a relaxed way to do 100kms. Except that what happened was by the time I started back on the road it was mostly the slower people left on the course. Instead of a group-ride it was a solo effort for the last 25kms - at exactly the time when you need the support the most. A couple of years later we did it again – this time we shared the load, and in the last 10kms I was just hanging on to my friend's back wheel. The cut-off was 4 hours, a pace of 25 km per hour, on that second occasion we pedalled in with less than 5 minutes to spare.

* * *

For the past few months Ken and I had been discussing how I was going to deal with his passing. Out of my mouth one day came "I'll train for Ironman whilst you fight Cancer, and you can be there on the start line to see me". "Can we have a deal on that?" Ken thought it was a great idea – but didn't share my belief that he would be on the start line.

By now it was becoming obvious that he would not get more than the 12 months predicted. Our plans to sell the house were shelved as I came to realisation that moving from Kāpiti would rob me of any social support structure.

Trying to hold him to a promise that he never made, I threatened not to do Ironman if he wasn't around. He said I would – and it would show me how strong I really was. I said I wasn't, and that I needed his support. He offered "to be there with me (in spirit) on the run", and then he added that my Dad would be with me on the swim. Dad had passed away 20 years earlier. He was a great swimmer, taking time out each lunchtime to swim in New Plymouth's outdoor pool. I asked who was going to be with me on the bike leg? Ken replied, "no one – you must train for that".

CHAPTER 21

Napier 2016 - Half Marathon

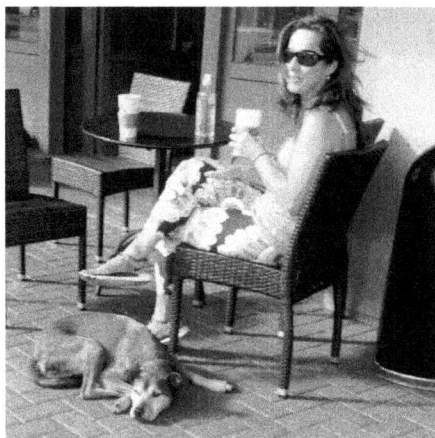

Ken, Buster and I travelled to Napier for a brief holiday. The Napier marathon was part of the Air New Zealand Runaway series. I had asked Ken if there was anywhere or anything he wanted to do before he got too ill. His answer was "no, nothing", my response was well that's good for you, but I would like some positive memories of this time. There were a couple of women from our training group heading to Napier for the Half Marathon, so under that guise we planned a long week-end away.

It was a shock to realise I would need to drive and take care of all the practical arrangements, that only used to happen when Ken had been intoxicated. I quipped that those years of drinking had prepared me for now - but it really wasn't at all funny. At least I still didn't need to fill the car with petrol. I left him and Buster at the motel while I went to the race. Only later finding out that Ken had taken Buster for a quick walk around the block - got lost - and arrived back just before me. I wasn't sure who I felt bad for but I knew I would need to step up and take responsibility for everything from now on.

* * *

14kms into the race I developed a pain in my knee. Not in a sense of something injured – the pain stopped when I stopped moving. But I could hardly walk on it. I concluded it was less painful and slightly quicker to run. And that's how I completed the event.

The pain had been developing in my knee for some time. I noticed that if I got out of bed in a certain way there would be a sharp pain. My mother suggested her acupuncturist. That seemed like a very good idea. I didn't have any more events planned. But I did want to continue to do the smaller triathlons. I had stated that I wanted to do the KWT every year for the next 20 years. The women participating in their seventies were such an inspiration, and it seemed a good way to carry "healthy" into those advancing years.

After discussing for some time all the ways in which the knee hurt, lots of needles were popped in and I lay quietly to let them do the work. We wrapped up the session and agreed I would return in a week to continue treatment. And then I said, "by the way my husband is dying".

No kidding that might have a lot to do with the physical problems I was again pushing to one side.

* * *

By now Ken had endured two brain surgeries and radiation treatment. Yet he was adamant that he would not be going down the chemo route. We had accidentally walked into the chemo room some weeks earlier and the shock stopped him from his usual bravado with the doctors and nurses.

Sadly, the time when I needed my mother and family support was when it disappeared. Her dementia rapidly worsened and I had taken responsibility for her dog. Jojo was not happy with the shared living arrangement and her first act of defiance was to poop in the middle of the spare bed. As I threw her out the backdoor by her collar, she knew she wouldn't be doing that again. It wasn't her fault later though when Ken was going for his first round of chemo, then I had to take the dogs with us to the hospital as it was going to be too long a day to leave them at home.

Regularly traveling from Kāpiti to Wellington Hospital took its toll. My temporary home-base was the Wellington hospital carpark. I would fill most of the day there, alternating between spending time with Ken, walking Buster, then walking Jojo, then heading to the hospital café for a coffee. Jojo gets car sick – and she took this opportunity to throw up in my handbag. At that point I honestly thought life couldn't get much worse.

* * *

What held it together was the 35 Day Detox Challenge. After unsuccessfully trying to fit the program into the running group as a 30-day

Challenge I had reclaimed it as mine, with its original 5-week (35 days) structure intact. Always starting a week before the new moon, setting an intention at the new moon, working the puzzle during the waxing moon, releasing and purging at the full moon, envisaging at better future as the moon wanes and finally resting.

Each cycle I was guiding friends and training buddies through the program and I was doing it for myself as well. I was armed with knowledge from the yoga training in philosophy, and I was prepared to approach transformation with as much diligence as I had applied to endurance training. There was no avoiding the "elephant in the room" as Ken's time was almost done and I would be embarking on a life without him.

My goal/affirmations for one cycle read like this:

- Move diet to anti-kapha so I'm light in the legs.
- Reduce stress at home.
- Enjoy the last of summer.
- Find ways to protect and shield my energy.
- Re-arrange the house for winter.

My reading list morphed into books that could help me understand mental strength; I was particularly drawn to biographies. It didn't take many books to realise that everyone has been through something significant, many people multiple times. The take-away was that yes our lives are full of crises but they don't need to be diminishing. They are life-changing, there are stories full of people finding the courage to go beyond their pasts as well as perceived limitations. I recall many years ago Madonna's answer in an interview as to why she had not written her biography yet; she said she hadn't experienced enough life yet.

The crucial book though was "The Tibetan Book of Living and Dying" by Sogyal Rinpoche. I had no idea what I was seeking in this book, but one of the yoga course instructors had reached out and pro-vided it as a reference. I downloaded it onto the Kindle. It became such an important book that I purchased the paper copy.

Although I felt helpless with the trajectory we were on, the book not only gave comfort, but it also more importantly gave me a sense of empowerment. Nobody avoids death. Yet I didn't know how to approach this important transition. Now I needed to learn.

* * *

As I saw my mother's narcissistic behaviour for what it was – it begged the question. Were Ken and I also caught up in the same web? On initial inquiry the answer could have been yes. When we met he was already established as a successful corporate executive and entrepreneur. He was nearly 20 years older than I. If I had dared use "me" in the previous sentence he would not have hesitated to correct me. But there is a very big difference between power and control. He was powerful but he wasn't controlling. I had chosen to defer to him and do anything to keep the peace throughout our relationship. Not because that was what he wanted – but it was my learned behaviour from childhood. When I was sure, or determined, and stood up to him – if the argument made logically sense - then he would easily defer to me and back my choice 100%. He wanted me to be my own person, but it was my responsibility to learn to be that person.

The regular acupuncture sessions were working. Perhaps too well as a lot of residual feelings of anger were surfacing. It didn't take much for me to kick-off at people and situations. Perhaps I might have thrown food on one occasion.

My anger was born out of stress and frustration. Frustration comes from a place of feeling dis-empowered. As I built the strength and self-confidence of the third chakra, I took responsibility for my actions, stood my ground on the issues that were important to me, and the anger fell away.

CHAPTER 22

Sri Lanka 2016 - YTT

Time on the YIN side!

There is a weird logic that takes over when you are faced with the "terminal" diagnosis. On one level you know that it will happen. On the other you don't want to push things forward by planning.

In that spirit I registered to learn about the YIN side of yoga. Up to this point I had been in the Vinyasa lineage, my own practice had recently strayed into a "restorative" approach. Firstly, as the endurance training became more intense and secondly, when the stress levels locked in the extreme position. Balance in life is achieved when you can be active when necessary and still when appropriate. Motion is initiated from the state of stillness, not from a moving platform. How many of us can pause and hold steady? I for one was in a state of perpetual motion.

Fifteen years earlier, when the bank had foreclosed on the house it had been tough to lose the very foundations of our life. Initially it was cool and exciting to move into an apartment in a new city, especially as we had the freedom to go where the business was. In hindsight I would say "careful what you wish for". Because a couple of years before that foreclosure I had envied our young marketing manager who packed up and followed her boyfriend to the UK to live. I wondered if we too could be free from attachments to pursue life. Anyway, I digress, this story is about why I was in perpetual motion. After a couple of years of moving around it was time to put down roots again. Come the weekends and Ken would have happily slept in – I couldn't. He asked when would I ever relax? I had a very simple answer – when we own a house again!

This was a flawed viewpoint. The truth is we are more effective when we start any action when we are rested. There is greater creativity, and you are more likely to intuitively nail the timing, ensuring that you have the Universe at your back.

We owned the house now, yet the feeling was the same – an acknowledgement that time was running out. Ken also felt it. It manifested in random calls to contractors to get things done. I could only watch helplessly as he called the electrician to come and fix a light switch. There was no explaining that it could have waited until there was another reason for the callout.

Some husbands may have arranged for flowers to be sent for Valentine's Day, or an anniversary. Mine decided to order over 20 cases of wine. The courier driver quipped that we must be about to have a great party. I stood open-mouthed as they were all unloaded into the hallway. I have rarely drunk wine since 2011. Ken's response to my question of "why", was "I don't want you to run out of wine". Clearly not for at least a couple of lifetimes. A year later I started selling the cases as the old adage rang true – "your assets eventually become your liabilities".

My journal entry from Wellington to Sydney in August 2016:

"I've never been a Qantas girl, give me Air New Zealand, Singapore Airlines or Emirates any day. Yet the feeling is the same. The antici-

pation of getting on a flight that will take off and go somewhere. It had been in the past a way of getting away – leaving something behind – but this time I'm not sure what I am running from. Maybe not, although the thought of just carrying on did seem impossible. So this is the reset.

Also this spiritual journey could be of help to Ken with his journey too. Reading the Tibetan Book of the living and dying it seems I can still help with my efforts. So I will stay the course with purifying my diet etc. with the hope that what I have done so far – and what I will do will help. The five negative emotions to work on – Pride, Anger, Jealousy, Greed and (and one I can't recall*)."

Note: The last one is "Attachment.

The past 12 months had been surreal. Initially life was borderline normal, before it was consumed with hospital appointments. The final episode was a slip on the concrete steps that eventually landed Ken in hospital and signalled the beginning of the end. A few days earlier was the first call to the local ambulance service as the seizures returned. The officers were incredible as they explained how they could help in the coming weeks.

Now I was calling because he hit his head while carrying a load of firewood. It was Friday afternoon; I called my friend and she dropped everything to come and get the dogs while I followed in the car to the Wellington Emergency Department. Seven hours later he was released and I drove him home. Ten days later and another seizure and another trip to hospital. This time they were not going to release him.

I credit this with being my finest hour.

This was the moment of reckoning for that old me – the one who refuses to throw up because she can't stand sickness. As a 6-year-old I ran away from home when my sister was vomiting. I also stole money from Mum's purse and went and got myself an ice cream from the dairy as compensation! Now I'm prepared to look after Ken in his final days. I argued with the Hospital staff who recommended that he go into the hospice system. I argued with my family who thought it was too much for me to handle. A sense of loyalty to Ken (and our relationship) was stronger than any argument – I was not going to concede. Once I won the battle, the medical system went into overdrive to ensure that all the support was put in place. Still it was a shock to comprehend that this time he wasn't coming home in the car with me. Rather in the ambulance.

Twenty-four years later Ken finally acknowledged that I was right about that very first argument we had. He now knew there was more to life than the here and now. He was receiving incredible downloads of spiritual information. We were able to sit night after night and talk with clarity that came directly from his higher self (Soul). Ego was gone. Though, not so much during the day – then he was his old self. I had given him a whistle to get my attention when I was out of sight. He blew it so much that I threatened to shove it up his backside if he didn't stop.

* * *

I arrived at Colombo airport and had arranged a car to take me three hours south to Fort Galle. In a daze I saw the name "Suzanne" and indicated to the driver that it was me. He took my bags and we made it to the car. As we exited the airport, he said it would only be a few minutes' drive. What? I thought he must mean something different. For few minutes I was confused, and then we pulled up at a local guest house. As we were debating where I thought we were going, the owner came out and berated the driver for not collecting the guest at the airport. Oops, I had got it wrong. I had my arranged driver's phone number. After much to-ing and fro-ing the two drivers agreed to meet on the airport expressway and swap passengers.

In Fort Galle I had chosen the place to stay because one of the other participants had posted on social media that she would be there a day or so earlier. As I walked around the fort I saw a lovely yogi with flowing hair and clothes, and wide brimmed hat. Bound to be, but after my luck so far it was way easier to turn around and scurry back to the room. Time to try again tomorrow.

Monday morning (Happy Birthday to me), I woke and got myself down to breakfast. I have always enjoyed hotel breakfasts on my own. I had an amazing Sri Lankan egg curry. I sat outside under cover of the balcony, the heavens opened up, and it poured with rain.

It was time to join the group for the car ride to the retreat. During the 3-hour trip everyone introduced themselves, excited for the week ahead etc. I sat there in silence. What could I say – "Hi, I'm Suzanne, it's my birthday and I'm 55 today, and my husband passed away a week ago."

My journal entry that morning:

"Bottling up my feelings as I really didn't want to say anything about Ken on my birthday. Maybe a mistake as I will definitely come across as closed off and perhaps even inauthentic."

It was comforting to see familiar instructors and students from previous teacher training modules, albeit in a different country. I had a separate bungalow and in this space it was safe to begin to process my emotions. Mostly that was in the shower at 3am, but strangely there were no tears. After the second day I was able to pull the instructor aside and tell him what I was going through. I didn't want the whole week to be about my situation, so it was kept low-key. I didn't need the course accreditation (now I had more teaching/training hours than most) but I did need the healing experience this training offered.

During the break some of the students practiced their "acro-yoga". Essentially this is partner yoga, and it consists of a base person and a flyer. I would have loved to try it but was not in a place to test up my level of trust in the Universe. Since then, I have tried and can confirm that my level of trust is pretty much non-existent – but if you can surrender to the safety of the base, the feeling is indescribable.

I noticed a pattern emerging. Each course had one pivotal reference book that came at exactly the right time and changed my life. And this training was no exception. The 2004 book "Eastern Body Western Mind – Psychology and the Chakra System as a Path to the Self" by Anodea Judith was it. I started with the Kindle version and later purchased a paperback copy as an ongoing reference. The heavy textbook on meridian lines, carried from New Zealand and never read, I left in the lounge upon checkout. Someone else needed it – not me.

I had become interested in the energy healing of chakras some years earlier. As I had cleaned up my eating habits in 2006 there was an expansion of awareness and I started to work with a couple of reiki healers. There was one at the Rhodes mall in suburban Sydney. She visited the organic health food shop once a month. I would seek her out when I was running on empty (yet again). I also found Doreen Virtue's chakra healing meditation online. Back then things were going great as I worked through the first chakra and its issues surrounding security and safety, then the second about acknowledging feelings, I loved the third about personal empowerment, but froze at the fourth chakra and the heart centre. Not going there yet.

Now I was feeling as if my heart was shattered. There was no avoiding the pain of the fourth chakra. Yoga teachers know of the emotional releases that can occur on the yoga mat. One minute you are fine and the next an emotional wave engulfs. Breathing is the only way through.

By day 4 the YIN practice was speaking to the emotions of FEAR (Kidneys), ANGER (Liver) and WORRY (Spleen). These are the natural reactions to the human condition. They are all filtered through the Heart and when they are present in excess, they rob us of the natural emotion of the heart – joy. In a moment of absolute clarity, I saw what I had been going through and I knew I was in exactly the right place at the right time. In that moment, as the instructor was playing his guitar, I could find the gratitude, and finally the tears.

As the training was wrapping up, I wasn't ready to come home. In an inspired moment, and with limited internet access, I rescheduled my flights and booked myself into a small hotel in Wellagma. I needed time out to process what had just happened. Sometimes things do just fall into place in a good way. The hotel only has a few rooms, they had been recently upgraded, my room had a stunning bathroom and the latest air conditioner. The owners went out of their way to make me feel at home. Their chef went to amazing lengths to provide stunningly healthy meals and decadent desserts. I walked on the beach each morning, smiled at the fishermen and even helping them with their boats. There was an Ayurvedic (traditional Indian healing) clinic about 20 minutes away by Tuk Tuk.

Wellagma is a tiny surf and fishing village on the south coast of Sri Lanka. It has an amazing sandy bay perfect for swimming and learning to surf. It also took the full brunt of the 2004 Boxing Day Tsunami. Twelve years on the devastation was still visible, and the collective grief of the many lives lost very much present. It was an exceptionally special time and triggered significant amounts of healing releases for me.

There was no concept of training for any endurance event – even though I did have the lingering promise of doing the Ironman – but that belonged to a different life. Instead I rolled out my mat each morning and did yoga. I downloaded random fiction onto my Kindle to read and generally gave myself permission to "not think". While I was in that state of nothingness the emotion poured out and the pressure valve was released a little.

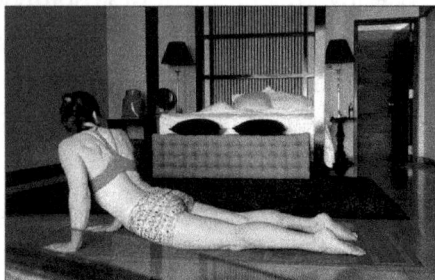

As the week came to an end – I had to fly home. Eventually everything needs to be faced and the reality is that you are never ready. So it just needs to be started. Which was fine until the final flight from Sydney to Wellington. It was the hardest of all. I didn't want to get on the flight and was crying my eyes out in the lounge before boarding. Then as we began to descend into Wellington I had a panic attack and locked myself in the toilet to calm down. Finally we landed and I was sitting in my seat. I was the last person to disembark that day. Do you know how long it takes to clear a plane? A very long time – but honestly not long enough.

CHAPTER 23

Napier 2016 - IronMāori Quarter Ironman (take 3)

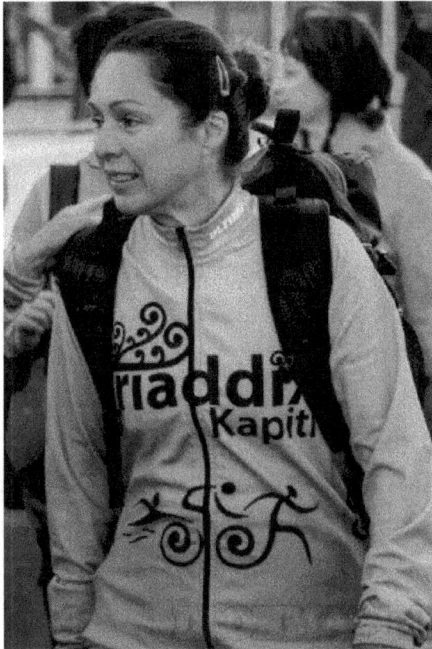

It was a very shaky return to racing. It had been over 18 months since I was on the start line of a triathlon. In that time my whole world had turned upside down. I considered not doing the Ironman – it seemed ludicrous to be embarking on such a journey of endurance after what I had been through. Ideally, I would have had 12 months training before the event – now I had 6 months. And my knee was still not right, that persistent twinge in the knee was diagnosed as patellofemoral pain syndrome (PFPS). I was energetically aware that it was about not moving forward in my life. In some twisted reality I figured that if I went ahead with the Ironman maybe the pain in my knee would go away.

This is a longstanding tactic I employ when faced with blocks in my life. Usually there is an internal dialog going that says I will do Y after X happens. When X doesn't happen and I find myself like the airplane circling the airport waiting to land in the fog - it is time to deploy the other strategy – make a start with Y and X will fall into place. Works every time!

I drove up to Napier a couple of days earlier with the intention of getting into the right headspace for tackling another triathlon. This was the first of the three races that would take me to the full Ironman. Quarter, Half, and then the whole shebang. The distances for the full Ironman are 3.8kms swim, 180kms bike ride and 42.2kms run. Say it quickly and you may not gag at the enormity of it.

I was almost at the destination, driving along the Havelock North by-pass when a stone hit the windscreen and created a crack through approximately two-thirds of the glass. I got to the Hotel shaking uncontrollably and completely lost it. Why did that have to happen – wasn't life difficult enough as it was? I gave up on the day, closed the curtains and went to bed.

The next day I called the insurance company and got the name of a local company to fix it. Problem was the glass wasn't in stock and wouldn't arrive until after I was due to return to Kāpiti. Could I drive with the crack – probably – that did nothing to calm my nerves. Sitting in the car I finally realised what had been strange about the incident. There wasn't another car on the road when it happened. Not in front, behind, or going in the other direction.

I planned to go shopping in Havelock North before registration. My parents had lived there for a few years, and I knew the area well. What I hadn't planned to do was go to see Dad's grave. I was the only one of the family that had not been. I had never wanted to visit. Now with the rawness of Ken's passing, it was time. I had no idea where his headstone was, and wandered around the cemetery for some time, hoping that I would stumble across it. Everything was so intense. There was a funeral service taking place in the grounds. Failing to find my Dad's grave I went back to the car defeated. I nearly drove away but as a last ditch I called my sister and asked for directions.

* * *

Back in 1998 when my father passed I didn't have time to grieve. Ken was negotiating an American investor to join the company and we had hired sales staff to expand. On the Friday evening there was a staff function to introduce the new team members, the following morning we were due to fly to Auckland to my first (and only) concert - Elton John and Billy Joel. During the party I received a call from my mother who broke the news that Dad suffered a mild stroke, he was in hospital but was OK. I suggested we come to Hawkes Bay – we already planned to be away for the weekend. Mum thought it wasn't necessary. Ken suggested we continue to Auckland for the concert and then fly to the Bay on Sunday to see Dad. It was just five weeks earlier that we had been there to celebrate his 60th birthday. The first birthday party he had ever had! I called our travel agent friend and asked him to change the flight in the morning. I sat through that concert in sheer panic. How could I be sitting there pretending to enjoy the performance? Despite what

Mum and Ken were saying my intuition was kicking in and I had a very bad feeling.

* * *

Registration takes place on the Friday before the triathlon. There was a gale-force wind and massive waves on Pandora pond. If it stayed like this it was going be a very tough day. I met up with the others and some of us called it quits on having a practice swim. Time for a quick bike ride along the shoreline to check that the brakes and gears were all working well. That was a non-negotiable pre-race routine – especially for out of town events - after the bike had been on the back of the car bouncing around there were often mechanical issues that needed to be dealt with.

The next morning we woke to a beautiful calm day with a bit of cloud. Chilly but it would get hot soon enough. I strapped up my knee - it was getting better – but still not right. It was good to be within a group, but I felt distant, somewhat removed. After everything I had been through it was hard to engage in a normal way.

My social media post courtesy of Facebook:

"All done!

Time to pack up and go. Very happy with my efforts this morning. The weather gods smiled and produced the perfect conditions. A few dramas along the way but I managed a positive attitude and pretty sure my time was faster than two years ago!

Oh god, next stop is twice the distance in 5 weeks' time. Still, we have time to celebrate first."

CHAPTER 24

Taupō 2016 - Half Ironman (take 2)

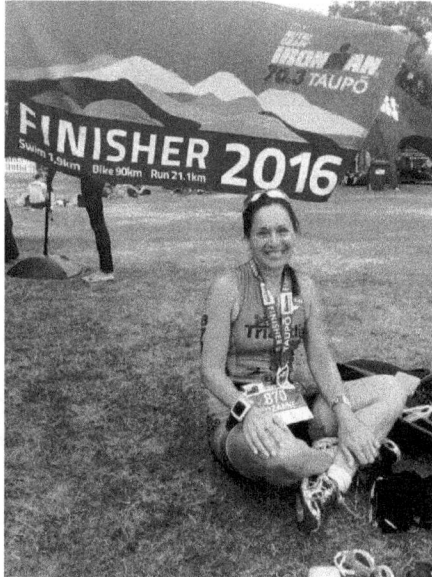

A good friend had advised me not to consume alcohol for at least six months after Ken's passing. I took it further and didn't eat junk food, processed food, or anything else that wasn't good for me. I was training to a program. This was the first time I had a coach for a triathlon. She knew me from KWT and, as a former Ironman, she was able to guide me in terms of the physical requirements, yet with empathy to know that sometimes I just couldn't stick with the schedule. In many ways training for this event gave my life structure and meaning.

With time on my hands, I started to build the weekly yoga classes. I now had a schedule that included early morning Vinyasa, mid-morning restorative, evening meditations, and the "crowd favourite" – hot yoga on a Sunday afternoon. I installed infrared heaters (as well as using the big gas heater) in the small 20 square metre studio. The combination of heat and humidity was perfect after a full weekend training, including those long Sunday morning bike rides.

Looking back there was a manic level of activity I engaged in. Not fuelled by caffeine, or a need to achieve anything. It was pure avoidance and a desire for numbness. Anything but feeling those feelings.

I had observed over the years that when I get tired (very tired) I tend to walk into doorways, drop things and generally become very uncoordinated. This became my benchmark as to when it was time to ease back on the training. Waiting for the energetic flow to return before digging deep again. The other indicator was a spike in my resting heart rate. These are great tools for endurance training, but they are also applicable to life in general. Catching that rise in cortisol before it affected my sleep was really important. This was not the time to be lying awake on my own. So much so that when the 2016 Kaikoura 7.8 earthquake hit just past midnight on November 14th, I popped both the dogs under the duvet and went back to sleep. If a tsunami came then so be it – we would float away on the bed. The next morning when I turned my phone back on there were missed calls and messages checking if I was okay.

One weird fallout from the grief was my sudden inability to sleep without two big pillows. The moment I put my head down lower than my heart I triggered a panic attack. It took several more years to progress beyond the panic attack and be okay with the sensation of feeling like I was going into a freefall. Yet from that small coping mechanism came significant neck and upper back issues.

Two years ago the Taupō Half Ironman was the "A" race – everything led to that moment. This time it was just a training race. Not competing for time – just to build the endurance – and prepare for the big day in four months' time. All I had to do was complete the event safely. The weather was good and it was one of those rare times when nothing phased me. Not even the fact that it would have been Ken's birthday that weekend.

All the big events have cut-off times for each leg. Generally the swim needs to be completed in 1 hour 10 minutes, after that it is time based. You can use the extra time saved in the swim to get through the bike – being back in transition by 12:30pm and finish the run before 4pm.

It was a practice run in terms of logistics, e.g. where I was staying, how to get gear to transition and what food and drinks I would be fuelling with. Including the night before, breakfast and recovery afterwards.

I had my blender with me – when I joked that I packed the car to go to an event – including the kitchen sink – it wasn't far from the truth. I had done some great training runs on that great kiwi classic – fish and chips. All the carbs in the chips, protein in the fish, and fat the night before worked for me. More healthy now was the homemade salmon, potato, egg and avocado salad I prepared. I struggled with digesting complex carbs at the best of times, particularly when it's a day of non-stop activity. Breakfast was my raw sprouted buckwheat porridge and banana with cacao nibs.

Along with the no alcohol and no processed foods, I wasn't drinking coffee. Instinctively I knew that my stress levels were through the roof and I was right on the limits with cortisol and adrenal function. According to my Garmin stats for the day I had burnt over 7,000 calories. Yum, that was a lot of food coming my way. The Indian Curry and Kingfisher beer were a perfect place to start refuelling.

At the end of the race I was heading to the UK for Christmas. Again, not ideal training preparation for Ironman. I didn't care. I knew that I couldn't face the holidays in Kāpiti. I questioned if I was doing a runner, or starting a new life? I was hoping for the latter. Hindsight is a wonderful thing. Clearly the answer to this question was the former. I was nowhere near the end of this journey.

CHAPTER 25

Road to Ironman 2017

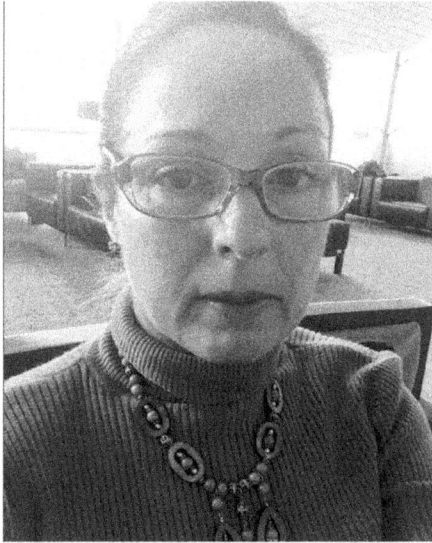

Training became the focus of my life. Each week I was doing between 12 and 18 hours of training, the preparation and recovery was probably the same again. I quipped it would have been easier to get a job. The reality was very different. I had no capacity to work. Even the simplest tasks seemed beyond my comprehension. My attention span was non-existent and even the slightest issue that came from left-field could spiral me out of control for days.

Once I was in the UK I relaxed, it was sufficiently far away from New Zealand. I did my sightseeing by running the streets, parks, and river trails of London. Come Christmas morning, my program had scheduled a half marathon training run around a small seaside town in Ireland.

I left early to give the family I was staying with some space, knowing I would be back in time to join them for the later part of the morning. No problem getting up, popping on woollen clothes, and getting out the door and down the drive. The plan was to run into town along the open road. We had driven it a couple of times and there weren't any significant hills. What could go wrong!

Well, when it is dark and there are no streetlights then quite a lot. That one streetlight at the first intersection let me get started. And then I was in a black abyss. I tried to find the reflector paint on the side of the road – but mostly there wasn't any. In tears from the shock of it all I considered turning around and going back to the house. But how pathetic would that seem, and I would still need to do the training run at some stage. I could walk and not fall in the ditch. But I was fit enough to run, why wouldn't I.

Eventually it would be light – I could wait for dawn. At that moment the sheer magnitude of how much my life had fallen apart hit me. I was on the other side of the world, at a strange house, trying to run on Christmas morning, and going to do an Ironman in three months. My internal dialog started listing all the "problems" with this story, but she was nowhere near as loud as before. I knew I was in the right place doing the right things and I would get through this test.

Eventually I started to run, a couple of cars went by heading into town. Nobody stopped and harassed me. Dawn broke and I made it to the outskirts of the town. I ran through town and out to the open road in the other direction. Back into town and down to the port, up to the farms, round the town and up the hill, and finally I had enough kilometres (14) to turn and run back to the house. All those kilometres on the open road – only eight – that had felt like hell at the start were quite pleasant on the return. Time for a shower – plenty of food and a day with new Irish friends in the pub and their homes. Something never to forget.

* * *

As part of stepping into this increased level of training I visited all the people who I perceived could help me prepare. The podiatrist to check the way I was running and to make sure I had the correct shoes. The physiotherapist to look at my lower back and core. The acupuncturist and Thai massage therapist. And finally the doctor to check bloods and get a new inhaler. This was the first inhaler I had had in over 20 years. It was clear by then that I was getting preventable cold induced asthma attacks in the water.

Really though I was trying to find some combination of external help that would put me back together. A way back to myself that would allow me to function on the back of the overwhelming emotion I was feeling. Eventually I had to pull myself together and learn to trust myself. After getting this far I would not be held hostage to the limits of my mind.

* * *

I became very good at training alone. Even clocking up over 100kms bike ride without leaving the 40km strip of the Kāpiti Coast. Starting with a 1.5km loop of Raumati South, followed by a 2km loop to the state highway, 6km to Raumati Beach, 10km to Paraparaumu, 12km to Otaihanga, etc., – and repeat in various combinations depending on whether I was feeling strong and motivated, or tired and ready to quit. These number patterns kept my brain engaged, gave me mini goals, and ultimately served to just keep me going.

CHAPTER 26

Taupō Ironman - Race Week

Driving up to Taupō I was in a good space physically and mentally. I had done all I could, and I recalled Ken's comment that Dad would be with me on the swim and he would be with me on the run. I felt confident with the bike itself – having chosen not to replace the bike – though I had given her an overhaul. She was sporting new racing wheels, gears and brakes. I knew that I wasn't a cyclist and that I would need all the hours available to complete the 180kms.

If I was steady, and the weather was favourable, then it was doable. I had let go of the "double plus an hour" potential time and was working on "completion" as the goal.

Leaving home, I packed everything I could conceive on needing plus a few extra things. My coach had commented that it was important to consider what you would put in to drop bags. I thought particularly about the one I would pick up towards the end of the run. I would be running in the dark and apart from food considerations I would need warmer clothes. As I picked up my favourite yellow long sleeve Nike top

I wondered what would cheer me up at that point. Colour is important - and yellow represents health and vitality – I would be needing that after a day of perpetual motion.

Freshly inspired I liberally sprayed the yellow top with my favourite perfume from Dubai days. It is called "Unforgivable" by the American Rapper Sean (P. Diddy) Combs. It is a scent that I had randomly found in duty free years ago – and I instantly loved it. What I couldn't comprehend was the name. What would be unforgivable? Why would I be unforgivable? I sought that perfume out everywhere I went for a few years. Picking it up in airport duty free stores, and very expensively in London, until I saw and purchased the last three bottles in Melbourne. Eventually a google search explained that Sean Combs stated that "a life not lived is unforgivable".

I was in the car, ready to back down the driveway when I stopped. I had the top/perfume for the run but I didn't have anything of Ken's. His spirit was going to be with me on the run – what could I take of his? A quick dash upstairs and I had his black onyx signet ring. He wore that for the 27 years we were together. Perfect. As I drove from Kāpiti I knew that I had time to take it to the jeweller in Taupō and have it resized. I would wear it in honour of him and our relationship.

* * *

There is a moment when you come north over the hill from Wellington and catch sight of Kāpiti Island. It takes your breath away. Although I had a generally negative attitude towards Kāpiti at this point, I appreciate that it is a special place, with special energy. It sits on the earth's ley lines, as do Napier and Taupō. Lake Taupō is the largest lake in New Zealand, lying in the middle of the North Island. The sight of this magnificent lake is equally emotional.

Now Lake Taupō brought me to tears. This was the comfort I was looking for. The Māori legend of the lake is that it is Aotearoa New Zealand's "beating heart". To me it felt like this was the moment of reckoning in the grieving process. I did not have a plan of what I would do after the race. All my attention in the past nine months since Ken had passed was to get to this point.

* * *

As part of my preparation I was very careful about the food I consumed in the three weeks leading up to the race. It was time to taper. That moment when all the hard work of training is done, it's time to ease back so that you are ready to race. Not just ready – excited and raring to go. For me tapering always had been a bit like when you go on holiday after working hard all year.

Initially the body is shocked and gets a bit derailed, then the "inevitable cold" sets in, finally it's time to recover as the reset button has done its job. Hoping that there are still days available to enjoy the break. That inevitable cold is when we finally ease up on all the collective stresses, our body says "hey now I can release some of the toxic load", and sure enough the nose starts to itch, then sneeze, then run. And the headache creeps up. And potentially the feeling that you have been hit by a bus. After a day or so these symptoms naturally disappear and there is a subsequent lightness of body and clarity of mind.

Nothing wrong with the detox/cold process if you don't buy into it being a problem. I turned my attention to ensuring that I was fuelling correctly. This was particularly true of hydration. My understanding was that hydration was something that you can get ahead of the curve on. Going into the race fully hydrated was within my control. Juices that include cucumber are my favourite as they are over 90% water and have the electrolyte minerals sodium, potassium, calcium and magnesium.

This recurrent experience of tapering helped with my understanding of the body's natural detox process and how we can use food and yoga to counter the physical effects. Although my primary focus was the physical, at this point I was deeply working with the emotional and mental bodies as well. Yogic philosophy explains these as the three manifest (tangible) representations of our Self. Beyond this our remaining bodies are unmanifest.

CHAPTER 27

Taupō Ironman - Race Day

I only had one strategy – keep going forward – and don't voluntarily quit. All the work I had done with my mindset through yoga and mindfulness was going to be tested in the sub-17 hours of swimming 3.8kms, biking 180kms, and then running the marathon of 42.2kms.

The back-up plan was to be pulled from the course. This took the decision away from me. I was free from the responsibility and that was incredibly liberating. If I couldn't continue then the medics and race officials could take that call. I was just moving forward. My mantras were "here, now, doing it" and "I am strength and courage in motion".

I knew of "tail end Charlie". And in many ways, I expected this is who I would be racing. In the 2014 Taupō Half Ironman bike leg I had watched tail end Charlie driving out to Reporoa as I was riding back into Taupō.

In this event would he pick me up and the day would be done? I didn't recall seeing him on the bike course during the day. So on the run I was on high alert. Towards the end of the event I asked my Coach where he was. Hilarious! Charlie was in front on me. The officials had presumed I would not finish and so they were tailing the guy in front of me.

Swim Course

The weather had been perfect in Taupō all week. Calm, warm but not too hot. Did I mention calm, as in no wind. The forecast wasn't so positive. High winds were due. Would they hold off until after the bike? Just after 4am I was woken by a gust of wind, and very strong winds ensued. They were not letting up any time soon. As we walked down to the start, the sight of large waves on the lake were a shock to us all. Over 200 people didn't finish the swim that day. Some of the Ironman distance people got caught up in the start for the Half Ironman and confusion about the cut-off ensued. It was gruelling but I put my head down and counted breaths. The waves were coming in sideways and all I could do was power my (stronger) left arm into each wave to stop myself from being pushed off course.

Bike Course

My fear with the bike has always been mechanical – ever since that first time at the Wellington Duathlon when the chain came off. The following fear rates almost as high – the possibility that I will crash. Still a crash in my mind was a legitimate way off the course and therefore I discounted that as a problem and hung onto the potential for needing to deal with a mechanical failure. After the madness of the swim, it was the wind that was an issue. Living on the west coast I was used to wind. Usually though we were riding into it. This time it was coming at us from the side.

All was going well, I was taking it slowly eating something every 20 minutes and drinking every 5kms. Playing with numbers is my thing.

Not only does it keep me focussed – it passes the time – and stops the negative self talk. It starts with the first 5kms. Then it's a matter of calculating the percentage of the course done, 5 of 180, a grand total of 3% under my belt.

After going through town and ticking over the first 90kms, my strategy was to stop at the next aid station and pick up my drop bag. Stretch a little, re-arrange things, reset for "just "a 90km ride. At this point I started to ditch things. The satisfaction of walking over to the bin and throwing out extra tubes, and heaven knows what else was amazing. Nothing was as good though, as later on the run when I went past a bin and undid my Camel belt/bottles and let the whole thing go. I had purchased that back in 2013 and it had been part of all my races. Did I need it to get to the finish line – no – therefore gone. I felt empowered to be releasing that which no longer served me and progressing towards the goal I had set.

* * *

The use of stimulants is just that – a desire to get energy where there is none. At the end of my endurance races all bets are off and passing through an aid station I reach for the caffeine and sugar. Where I wouldn't normally consider coke as a drink this is the time to grab whatever will get me to the finish line.

We do that in life too. Using caffeine (or even superfoods like maca and cacao) to excite the physical self to achieve a goal (even if the goal is just to get through the day). That energetic debt needs to be repaid at some point. We can defer it for days, weeks, months, years - but eventually it needs to be repaid. Now doesn't that sound a bit like our relationship with borrowing money. The burden of debt is exhausting and a never-ending spiral that keeps us pedalling. It is way easier to come off the stimulants of our own accord. Otherwise the body calls time and enforces rest.

Another way to hack this system is to look for any statement that starts with "I'm tired ...", of someone's behaviour, a situation, feeling a certain way. That's the cue to ease up and bring yourself into balance. Self-care and self-nurturing will restore the equilibrium to the situation.

CHAPTER 28

Taupō Ironman - Run Course

It was a shock to see my shadow as the sun was setting. I was leaning to one side. That was weird – I didn't feel like that, I thought I was straight. I wasn't in pain – was it my mind playing tricks with the angle of the light. Then one of the other competitors ran past and asked me if I was okay. Yes I was fine. Was having to walk a bit – but hey ho – that was me. I was calculating that I could walk the whole distance and still make it before midnight. I had arrived back from the bike leg at transition at 5:15pm, the bike cut off was 5:30pm.

That gave me 6 hours 45 minutes to do the marathon. Very doable. If I kept moving forward. The course was three loops of 14kms. It was going to be a long evening but the wind had dropped and there was a beautiful sunset to enjoy. I swapped my sun visor and sunglasses for my yellow long sleeved jersey at the halfway mark. Now it was dark and some of the supporters had set up BBQs and mini street parties. The offers of a cold beer as I passed were very tempting.

With less than 7kms to go, it was a matter of getting back to the finish line. I was at the furthest point in the course. Speaking to my coach we crunched the numbers yet again. Yes, if I kept going at this pace I would be in okay. A physio joined the conversation and it was agreed that I could take five minutes for him to strap my back. Climbing on the table was such a relief. I could have just called it quits there and then. Perhaps an ambulance back to town? Yeah, that wasn't going to happen. All that was wrong was that my back muscles had seized up on the left side. Most likely from the extra effort of swimming into those waves earlier in the day, and then exacerbated by gripping onto the aero-bars on the bike. Oh, she with the great core strength was being let down by her back muscles.

By now my coach was very insistent that I got off the physio's bed and keep moving. Those extra few minutes had been used and I needed to get moving and keep moving. The women from Kāpiti were with me all the way. As we went along the lakefront, I was joined by some of the local firefighters. They were in their kit and had come across the road from the station to give a bit of a morale boost to the last finishers. Clearly, they are trained to take people's minds off the present disaster. With questions such as why are you doing this? What is keeping you going? Do you say anything to keep you motivated?

That was a good question. I was repeating a couple of mantras all day. One of my favourites was "I am courage in action".

Most of the spectators had long gone as I shuffled up the road. Then I came to the metal barriers that signalled I was entering the finishing-chute. You would think at that point I would be motivated to finish. But here was that "close enough is good enough" moment. My body sagged and I couldn't move forward. Out of the mouth of a very mild-mannered gentleman came the directive "you're not f@#king giving up now". I didn't even question that order – I was back on my way. I could hear my name coming over the loud speaker system. The count down was on to cross the finish line before midnight. It was surreal and a bit like the story of Cinderella at the ball. I have absolute clarity of the last three minutes ticking by as I made my way along the carpet. However the tank was truly empty and all I could do was what I had prophesied - keep putting one foot in front of the other.

I was delivered to the recovery tent in a wheelchair. I guess it was expected that I would be in a bad way physically. A check of my heartrate and a few questions later, I was told "No you are fine – maybe a couple of Panadol!"

Ah but can I walk? Yes, right over to the massage table.

What I put on Facebook:

"Where's the smiley face for when you are so overwhelmed you have no idea how to respond to the situation. It was always going to be an epic journey, and I did say it might not be pretty, but it would be done. Little did I know how ugly it would get.

I had a great swim and came out feeling pretty pleased with myself. 1.30 was what I thought was possible on a calm day and I'd done it in a washing machine. The bike I just had to get done. The winds were just like almost all my training rides (minus the rain) and I struggled but ended at 8.35 with 15 minutes spare. So I thought 6.30 for the marathon was doable.

My body thought otherwise and with 12km to go one of the physios strapped me ribs to hips to try and straighten me up. So much for my strong yoga core! The rest is now history.

Coach Lynley and the Triaddix support crew more than had their work cut out in the last hour. I am so grateful to them all.

It wasn't an option to stop. It was always about me and the cut-off times. But there's close and then there is surreal.

What has blown me away the most is the outpouring of support from everyone. It's so incredible and scary at the same time. Thank you so much for the love.

No I will never do such a thing again."

CHAPTER 29

Publicity

This was my 15 minutes of fame whether I wanted it or not. I had not considered what it might be like to cross the finish line at an Ironman event. Let alone be right on the cut-off like Cinderella's coach turning into a pumpkin at midnight. My visualisations hadn't gone there, and I was quite happy that most supporters had packed up and gone home hours ago. It was embarrassing enough to have had the fuss about finishing at midnight, let alone being wheeled into the recovery tent.

As we got back to the hotel room my friend received messages that the finish was being shared on social media. My phone was switched off – and it could stay that way.

We had planned to stay in Taupō on the Sunday and drive back Monday. I even had tickets to go to the dinner – why not milk the event for all it represented. Now all I wanted was to pack up and get out of there. I needed to be back in the safety of my home. Fuelled on caffeine, I actually felt good when I got up on Sunday and not phased when there was a major detour on the Desert Road.

When I woke at home on Monday morning I felt like it had all been a nightmare. The sugar and caffeine had left my system and I was numb. A friend called and within a minute I was crying my heart out as the unspoken question finally came up. Ken promised me he would be there on the run – why wasn't he? I had imagined some spiritual moment where I would feel his support and be inspired to continue. Feeling devastated, my friend (one of the few people in the circle that had personally known Ken) drove by after the school drop off. As I continued to repeat my question, she answered it for me. "He said he would be there – he didn't say he would help." And that was the truth right there!

Then came phone calls to see if I was interested in doing an interview.

With the publicity also came the controversy – was it legitimate that I finished? Should I have been given the medal? Was I an Ironman or not? I didn't know – all I wanted to do was hide. Should I be ashamed of what happened. Certainly I didn't feel proud of the achievement. Somehow it had been spoilt. There was never a thought of having the usual post-event dinner. I was going to be on the course way into the night. But the next day, we usually all got together and went through the highs and lows of the day. Some of the women decided to go shopping, and even that tradition of getting together to debrief the day just fizzled to a couple of us. Nothing felt right about what had happened.

I was receiving messages from people that knew me who had been watching the live feed about the event. It had been emotional. The reporter came to the house for the interview. He asked to see the medal, I looked blankly at him. I had no idea where it was. I politely declined to have a photo with it. Later I found it in amongst the dirty laundry.

A few days later an email arrived from Mike Reilly, the "Voice of Ironman". He had been calling the finishers that day and had come down to meet me on the finishing carpet. He concluded the message with "Suzanne Stokes, you are an Ironman". I wasn't going to get any more validation than that. Best shut up and move on with my life.

What life though? If anything it felt like a game of snakes and ladders. Each time I progressed up the ladder and thought I was doing okay, the dice rolled again, and I was sliding down the snake. It was less than a year since Ken passed.

After Ironman I took a break before thinking it was time to take the 35 Day Detox business to the next stage. I wanted to do a series of talks on the various subjects that make up the Challenge, and my idea was to start with "the ancient art of Feng Shui". The painters were contracted to give a fresh coat of paint to the house, the invites went out to the workshop, and the acceptances rolled in.

It is a standing family joke that I cannot leave anything as it is. I constantly re-arrange the furniture. Seriously I sit down at a restaurant and re-arrange the contents of the table so everyone can connect without obstruction; walk into a hotel room and move things around and put away all those annoying pamphlets and promo materials. Apparently, I wasn't very old when I shut the bedroom door and managed to lift one single bed on top of the other on my way to turning the room around 180 degrees. In later life I was using the principles Feng Shui principles to support the changes I was making in a particular area of my life. I used colour and shape to bring the rooms (and my life) into harmony.

On the day of the workshop, it all fell apart again. I wrapped up the talk at 4:30pm, put the jug on for a cuppa, gathered some firewood to make a fire. The phone rang. The dogs were in Otaki at a vet nurse's property. I knew 9-year-old Buster had not been well for a couple of weeks but the local vet had done tests and concluded it must have been something he ate on the beach. Now I was being told that he had internal bleeding and I needed to choose between emergency surgery or letting him go. I jumped in the car and drove the 25km to Otaki. My cell phone went and the nurse said she didn't think they could wait for me to arrive to make a decision. I called it that we would let him join Ken but asked that they wait until I arrived.

One of the conversations that Ken and I had at the end was regarding our pets. He said that we have one animal that is our companion here on earth. That these partnerships have formed over many lifetimes. I asked if Buster was his animal, and he said yes. I looked at Jojo and asked if she was mine. He didn't answer, instead telling me that her name was previously "Rosie".

I held Buster while he was given the sedative. He should have drifted to sleep but he was fidgeting in my arms. They gave him more sedative, and the nurse suggested she hold him. He still would not settle. I couldn't take it. Then it dawned on me. I said, "give him back to me, he wants one last belly rub". I rubbed his belly. Then all the energy left the room, it was icy cold and still. Buster was gone too.

If I thought the grief was unbearable before it seemed as if this was way more intense. It took everything, rolled it into a big ball, and threw it at me. Post event depression is a thing. After the euphoria of a major event, then it would be natural to experience a corresponding dip. Blast, I'd missed the high and was just spiralling into the low. All the issues surrounding grief kicked in.

- Yes the loss of a partner.
- Also the loss of a shared future.
- The loss of a business.
- My lack of identity as a businessperson was a continued struggle.
- Alienation from my family due to my choices.
- And then I felt the betrayal of a partner who even after 27 years had chosen to exit stage right.

In hindsight I could see Ken's illness came at a time when I could see the connection between food and health. Not to say I ever thought I could save him with green smoothies and kale salads. But I did think he could have tried. "No", he said, "he was tired, and it was his time, and he was ok with that." "No, my feelings on the subject did not make a difference." Eventually I learned to respect that we all are ultimately responsible for ourselves. We cannot fix each other.

* * *

I was vaguely aware that my father had experienced depression throughout his life. Not at the time, only some years after his passing. It had been clear to me for many years that my mother also experienced it. Now I needed to label the patterns that were showing up time and again in my life. I knew anxiety, it had been a companion for many years. I had faced fear head on and dealt with that. But there was something deeper at play that I couldn't name.

Another realisation came regarding the connection between food and my emotions. I hadn't stopped eating since finishing training and the Ironman event in March. My body was so depleted, it craved the fuel for recovery – however all those carbs were playing havoc with my emotions. All the walking I had done that night had caused blisters on the soles of my feet. Like a snake I was literally shedding my old skin.

If the problem was food, then I concluded the solution would lie there too. Kitchari is an Ayurvedic recipe that is nourishing and helps to bring the body back into balance. Consisting primarily of rice and beans it is a complete food (carbs, protein and fats) suitable for all constitutions. I cooked up huge pots of the stuff and that's all I ate for a month. My taste for food and life returned.

I used the meditative tool of sun-gazing to tackle the depression. Watching the sun set each evening, often photographing the amazing

Kāpiti sunsets, and forcing myself up early the next morning. Walking the 1.5km to the river to watch the sunrise, planting bare feet in the middle of the stream, seeing the light change as the sun moves closer to the horizon.

Experiencing the rhythm of the sun daily connects us to the realisation that there will be another day, and change will eventually come through.

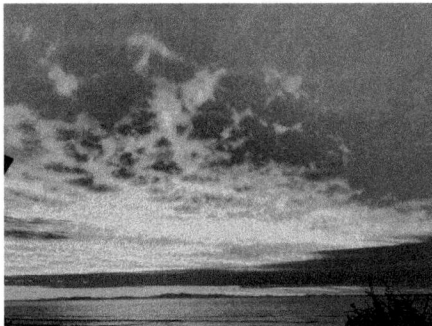

CHAPTER 30

Bryon Bay 2018 - YTT

The state of vigilance I experienced during Ken's illness could be summed up by the fact I purchased an Apple Watch just so I would be instantly contactable by him (or the medical team) at any moment. This state is difficult to recover from. It takes time to convince the mind and body that it can relax.

All those yoga classes were helping to keep me centred. I thought I couldn't get enough yoga. Until the Friday I approached the fifth class of the day by falling asleep for a 20-minute nap and was woken two hours later by one of the students knocking on the door. Good thing it was a meditation class, I didn't wake up – literally channelling the session in an almost sleep-state.

* * *

Buster's passing hit me hard. Jojo and I were desolate. We walked around the house not knowing what to do. I couldn't cheer her up and then another of those fated moments intervened. A post went on Facebook about a 5-month-old puppy that urgently needed re-homing. The sadness of a puppy sitting in a chair in the vet's office without a home was too much to bear. We will embrace our own suffering but when it comes to the defenceless that is a whole different world of sadness.

Sadness is a result of a perceived punishment of some description and is one of the basic human feelings. I could barely look after myself, yet I sent a message to my friend anyway asking if it was meant to be? "Was the puppy destined to be mine?" Could I address that sadness within by moving beyond the victim mentality and choose new life that involved caring for another?

Of course it was, his name was Beau; Jojo and I did the meet and greet. I asked for a sign from the Universe and when we got back to the vet carpark there was a dog the spitting image of Buster. Jojo thought it was great having a puppy in the house for about 24 hours and then she wondered when he was going home. I thought because he was about the same size as Buster that he was fully grown. Everyone kept saying – no – look at the size of his feet. When I found one of his puppy teeth on the bed I realised he was still a baby - just a very big one.

* * *

I desperately wanted to find my new tribe. I was determined to see Ken's passing as an opportunity, a chance to be like the Phoenix and rise from the ashes. Mostly I was adamant I was not going to be like my mother. I was 54 when Ken passed, Mum was 58 when Dad died; and whether I liked it or not there were significant parallels in our lives.

We learn as much from what we don't resonate with, possibly more. Which may explain why the stick (negative) is more effective than the carrot (positive) in providing motivation in the story of the getting the donkey moving. And it says a great deal about our relationship with Self in that we are conditioned to prefer punishment to reward to facilitate change.

Yet everything I touched, and thought was my way out the other side of the grief, fell apart. Some of things I tried were:

- Partnering with another yoga teacher to provide the Detox Challenge. Had I not learnt from the previous attempt to partner with a running club? She went on to create a series of retreats without ever inviting me back.
- I joined my friend in Europe for a trip only to find it was not for me.
- I signed up with a network marketing organisation (actually two), only to realise that wasn't for me either.
- Finally I joined my family for a holiday in Hawaii, only to learn it wasn't my sister's idea that I was there. That felt like a re-run of how my mother was included because it was expected rather than desired.

I didn't plan any further endurance events; after Ironman I desperately needed to rest, but deeper than that was my feeling again that they were a distraction and a waste of time. They had served a very important part of my transformation but now I wondered if I needed to move on.

My question after a couple of months was "when can I take Beau for a run". The standard answer is a dog will be ready to run short distances between 6 and 12 months. When their bones have stopped growing. My friend had a clearer message, "at your pace I don't think it will matter!"

* * *

Running with Beau was a joy from the outset. I enjoyed going out into the park, on the beach, and along the roads. The wisdom of Satyong Mipham came back to me. I felt I had progressed through the Tiger and Lion phases and was at the Garuda stage – running as a meditation. This third stage is where you can enjoy the surroundings, not caught up in the physical effort of running, or distracted by the stories of the mind. Able to appreciate the moment, be present with the freedom and power of running as a natural human activity. The final stage is one where you are running for some purpose (a goal greater than you, maybe raising funds for charity).

Apart from running my meditation practice at this point was non-existent. I found it difficult to sit and meditate, the best I could do was spend time in the garden. Frequently overwhelmed with emotion I forced myself outside for at least 20 minutes a day no matter the weather. Determined not to return to the house until I had shifted my perception of my present situation. The house itself was beginning to feel like a prison. The beautiful cedar blinds acting as bars across the window. I was finding myself driving to the supermarket – not for groceries – but to sit in the carpark and get distance from home and my life.

Reading "The Accidental Tourist" by Anne Tyler summed it up for me. I'm not sure if one particular scene made it into the movie. But when the main character describes an idea of how to arrange the bed to save washing sheets, I totally resonated. I knew I was in trouble. All my actions were calculated to do as little as possible. Looking after two dogs, a house, trying to establish a business, and showing up in the world was too much. Washing my hair, taking a shower, caring for myself, became secondary to getting through the day.

* * *

As we fit into social structures we conform to pre-conceived roles. As we meet new people, we ask questions in order to determine how they fit into that view. Any answer will suffice. We all have multiple roles, and the easiest way is to answer based on what the person wishes to hear. My experience is that despite this categorisation most people are not really interested in who you are, or what you have done. This is liberating in that you can opt out of defining yourself through other people's eyes. The most important viewpoint is that of you looking at you. First though it is necessary to address the "loss of identity" and be prepared to own the blank canvas.

Beau was already named by the time he came to me. It is a French word and the masculine meaning is "handsome" – what a perfect name for a beautiful boy. When I received his papers I found he was born on February 14th 2017, Valentine's day. That was the first without Ken, so I took Beau as his valentines present for me. And if he wasn't special enough in my eyes, one of my friend's young daughter drew a picture of Beau and coloured him as the Rainbow. I often see rainbows as confirmation of being on the right path – it's been a thing of mine since Ken passed. So now he is nicknamed Rain-Beau.

* * *

To further my studies of the philosophy behind the science of yoga I headed to Bryon Bay in NSW, Australia. The prerequisite reading this time was the "Jaya – an illustrated retelling of the Mahabharata" by Devdutt Pattanaik. Essentially a tale of dharma. Dharma is the concept that we all have a destiny and it is our responsibility to find it and follow it. Not to follow someone else's plan for you.

That raises a big question about "destiny vs free will". I believe that both are at play. We have a destiny that is pure potential. These are opportunities for experiences and lessons over a lifetime. Sometimes the destiny is to do something that will create a learning opportunity for another (no it's not always about me). At all times there is free will as to how to act. Choice is the action that creates free will. Choice is the point at which we enter the dialog between destiny and free will.

On page 53 of the JAYA there it was. I jumped up and let out a scream. I had known IT all along but never seen the story of astrology written in any of the ancient texts.

It comes from the story of "Pandu" the father who lived a happy life in the forest; he said, "years of celibacy and meditation in the forest have given me great knowledge." He passed the knowledge to his son. That son was Sahadeva who "realised the future could be deciphered if one observed nature carefully." In South India Sahadeva is renowned as the master of astrology, face reading and all other forms of divination.

All the knowledge is written in the stars. My interest in Astrology was not some random hobby - bingo – it was part of the story, one of the pieces of the puzzle. This is my belief that the guidance system is there for us to use. For me astrology is a way to put life into context. It is the instruction manual for what is taking place within the individual and the collective, but no one else seemed to have the same opinion. I intuitively understood now that I just had to keep growing until I matched up with those that did.

This interest started after my father passed away in 1998. Things were not going well in the business, and some months later I required surgery for ovarian cancer. I felt I was missing a part of the puzzle. On paper we were doing everything right – but nothing was turning out well. I purchased Joseph Polansky's astrology book for 1999. He highlighted the good money days, difficult days, etc. Was it the power of intention or something more? Statistically those were the days sales would happen, or money would finally arrive. Knowing that wasn't enough for me though, after buying the books each year I started to use the internet to correlate what was happening with the astrology to match up the days. Very soon I was tracking the moon's phases too.

After more than 20 years I had an unshakable belief in the connection. Pieces of the puzzle were falling into place. Now I felt like I was actually a yogi. Hey, I had all the pairs of lycra pants to prove it. I knew the drill of what to take to a yoga teacher training retreat. At the last minute I was given an option of a room to myself. Yes I'll take that. When it came to doing backbends, handstands and all the Instagram-seque poses, I was just left wondering why I was there.

I was shocked to read my journal entry from a family holiday in Hawaii at the end of 2017:

"Feet in the sand daily. Trying to stay connected to humanity and this life. Because there is a strong desire not to be part of it. Which is why I think this time I really do need help. That lack of connection is getting me down. Yes at a superficial level I can engage. I got it so wrong that I was welcome. Maybe being home with the dogs is the best thing I can do. There's a new moon coming – just as this holiday comes to an end. And it will be time to reflect on 2017 and what I want from 2018."

Continuing the theme of things coming into my life when they were most needed. This teaching module included instruction on the various yogic breathing techniques (pranayama). Grief is energetically stored in the lungs. All those years of allergies, hay-fever and asthma had reduced my lung capacity. Now it was time to clear them.

In my mid-twenties a book that impacted me was by the actress Shirley MacLaine. It shaped my belief that we have more control over our body than my education had suggested. In one scene she describes being on a mountain and very cold. Her teacher shows her how to use breath to warm herself. In this current millennium we have Wim Hof as the ultimate guide on the body breath connection.

Breath can be used to heat, cool, calm or excite. I was particularly interested in the Nauli Kriya. In yoga kriya is a set of actions done to achieve a specific result. Nauli is a breathing technique to stimulate the diaphragm, and digestive areas. Each morning on the yoga mat I would practice three sets to stimulate the diaphragm and (literally and metaphorically) cough up all my stored grief.

CHAPTER 31

Kinloch Sprint Triathlon - Did Not Finish (DNF)

Once more there were a group of women from the local triathlon club traveling to Taupō to do the Kinloch Triathlon in February.

For the past few months I had opened my house to international travellers via HelpX, an online barter system matching travellers with hosts. A friend had suggested that it might be a way to get some assistance with the upkeep on the house. But it was so much more than that. From the moment the first young French woman arrived, I knew I had found connection and purpose. My dogs loved having people to stay. They got numerous additional beach walks and non-stop attention. Each evening we gathered round for a shared dinner, talked about their experiences of New Zealand and their homes and families. We often discussed their reasons for travelling, what they wanted to do with their lives, and I offered advice on the changes they could make. More than one once I had messages from their parents who were glad to know their son or daughter was safe in a foreign land.

One time a lovely South American couple stayed. They house-sat while I was away and looked after the dogs. The day after they left I tripped on the rocks on the beach and broke my toe. It was only a hairline crack but enough to stop me in my tracks. I was physically incapacitated and needed help, just when it wasn't there anymore! I took it badly, like another universal slap in the face. Here I was trying to make progress, putting myself out there only to have the carpet ripped out from beneath my feet. Taking the remaining supply of Ken's painkillers, I hobbled up the beach daily with a piece of driftwood as a walking stick. My neighbour bailed me out - her husband could walk Beau for me. I crawled up and down the stairs for a few days and finally worked out that if I wore my bike shoes I could move around the house.

Right here in that story, was the extent to which I was prepared to go - in now not seeking external help – and feeling that I was on my own on this journey.

Two weeks later cycling and swimming was fine, training could resume. Although I couldn't push off from the side of the pool for another two months. Damn not learning those tumble-turns as a teenager.

This time I was prepared for the hills on the Kinloch bike course. I always enjoyed the swim in Lake Taupō, what I wasn't sure of was whether I would be able to run (or even walk) the 5kms to finish. Perhaps it didn't matter.

The swim start was from the shore. A few steps, and then a duck dive or two to get underway. As I didn't want to hurt my foot on the uneven ground I chose to stay back and cautiously entered the water. It meant I was going to end up swimming through people but I wasn't too concerned about that now. I was developing an instinct of finding the right swim-line to take, and I was trusting more that things were okay.

But something went very wrong, I found I couldn't lift my arm overhead. If, at the outset you don't adjust your wetsuit for the range of motion that can cause restriction, but it wasn't that. Treading water

I tried to comprehend what had gone wrong. I looked at my hand and saw Ken's ring – I had been wearing it since Ironman. Instinctively now I knew it had to go. I took it off, ducked my head under water and let it drop to the bottom of the lake. The water was so clear that I was able to watch it drift downwards for some time. Then I popped my head up, sighted the first buoy, and started to swim – I was back in the event.

It rained throughout the race, but I was smiling because that race was won for me in the first few minutes of the swim. Out on the bike and up and down the hills – passing like a pro – not concerned about the wet roads. Run shoes on, out of transition and along past the spectators. I was running cautiously to see how the toe would hold up. The moment I was outside the crowds there was a slight incline. And that was it – pain. This time I wasn't planning to push through, I walked and, finding the track back to transition, I handed in my transponder and went to find the others.

I thought I was okay – we were now watching the Pro and Elite racers on their bikes. In the wet I could see an accident just waiting to happen. Sure enough there was a slide and I watched in horror as the collision occurred at the roundabout. I burst into tears – and couldn't stop – my friend took me back to the house. Everything that had transpired in the last six months came up for release.

What if we could turn the healing back on itself? All the endurance events had one thing in common. At the end there was a release of some description. The tanks were emptied, and the sludge of my life exposed to face. The practice of yoga mimics life, we face our physical shortcomings, mental conditioning, and emotional pain right there on the mat. My lightbulb moment was tying these together, turning 180 degrees and deepening the yoga to clear the pain. Adding a issue-focussed yoga practice to the toolkit to access the hidden parts of self – to consciously bring them to light to heal them.

It was time to get a Tattoo.

Both my mother and Ken were adamant that tattoos were something to be avoided. My position was if there was a good reason then it would be my choice. Now it was time to honour Ken. I felt that having a permanent reminder would signify my carrying his energy within me.

I knew what the tattoo would be. It was the Eagle flying south over Kāpiti Island. Kāpiti Island, ever present on the horizon, the benevolent green dragon watching and protecting us. Regarding the Eagle, on the morning of his passing I had captured a photo of the island as the sea turned green, and I saw the shape of the bird flying south in the clouds over the island.

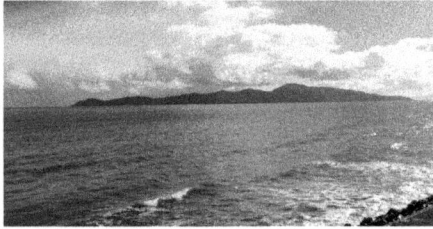

It reminded me of the native Indian myth of the Eagle and Condor. As the ages change there will be a moment when the Eagle flies south to meet the Condor. The end of the masculine dominance and the rising of the feminine energy. Both energies will be present equally. Each person will be whole and complete within themselves. A new approach to the world will be birthed, resulting from the integration of the masculine and feminine principles within.

Throughout our lives together the number "8" was present in all the significant events. Right from the first time we went to lunch together 8/8/1988 to the day I flew to Bali in 8/8/2015 and his passing on 8/8/2016.

I expected there to be pain – it was a rite of passage after all - a release of the emotional pain alongside the physical. As I drove away from the tattoo parlour I questioned if I had done the right thing or made a monumental mistake. I wondered if Ken would approve. Coming towards me was his favourite car. I pulled over to the side of the road and spluttered something between a laugh and a cry. From a distance my tattoo looks exactly like the Bentley logo. He had the last laugh – yet again!

* * *

That first DNF felt like a metaphor for my life as I was struggling to gain any traction and forward momentum. Ken and I had talked about the 35 Day Detox program, and he was adamant that it was going to be my focus. He was very proud of the recipe book and was even prepared to cook "healthy" from it. He had spent hours proofreading the manuscript. One of our ongoing jokes was regarding my inability to learn a second language and his retort was always that I was still trying to learn English.

I questioned the emerging pattern of making efforts in the business, and then pulling back. Did I lack motivation? No, I was very passionate about the principles that made up the program and it was really the only time I found any enthusiasm in a conversation. Was this another layer of self-sabotage? I thought I had worked my way through that limitation. Was I feeling guilty for building a life? Again, I didn't think so. Could it be about not finding my voice yet? Bingo, fifth chakra (located at the throat) stuff.

The Chakras have specific energy vibrations – the includes sound but also colour. Blue is the colour of the fifth chakra. It didn't take much – a quick look in my wardrobe sufficed. True there was nothing that was blue – hardly a hint. I favoured the reds, oranges, and browns of the first and second chakras. This was where most of my healing had taken place. I'd added yellow as I worked with the third chakra, and green was prevalent as I moved through the healing of the fourth – heart chakra.

It's my working theory that the reason coffee is such a popular ritual is that is essentially grounding us via the first chakra. Seeing the deep brown hue of the drink, stopping to saviour the bitter flavour, it is a moment that helps to bring all the pieces of life together. Then the caffeine kicks in and over-stimulates that body and mind – but that is another issue.

White includes all the colour spectrum; black is the absence of light. In New Zealand we mostly wear black, all the time. It's almost a national uniform. I was shocked to start traveling and see that wasn't the case in other parts of the world. In 2007 I set myself a challenge to not buy anything black for a year. No black shoes, handbags, or clothes. My wardrobe morphed into something very different – as did my life. Later I came to understand that wearing black absorbs the energy of the room. Great if you have some priestly aspiration to take on others' suffering. I didn't, so deliberately chose what to wear accordingly. Plus, when I instinctively reach for a particular colour, I get immediate insight as to where my emotional body is right now.

Now it was necessary to consciously choose something blue for the fifth chakra. Even if it starts with a t-shirt, which is exactly what it was.

The Throat chakra is about speaking your truth; this requires the stability of the lower chakras to speak up. Without that stability the voice is that of bullying, untruths, and manipulation. It is also about the ability to listen and hear the truth from others.

CHAPTER 32

IronMāori Quarter Ironman 2018 - Did Not Start (DNS)

In some moment of hubris, I thought that I can do both the Queenstown marathon and the Napier Quarter Ironman within two weeks of each other.

My thoughts were: "It will be a bit of cross-training and I get to hang out with lots of training buddies." It is true that time spent on the bike and swimming is good for keeping you in shape. But I realised I couldn't focus on both. I had to admit that age does play an important factor in the training. With what training is possible, but more so the amount of recovery time that is required.

Is this the part of the story where there is some great spiritual awakening? Yes and no. No in that there weren't angels coming down from on high heralding the start of something new. I envied my friends who could connect with their guides, and had a connection with Gaia (Earth), and the unseen realms. This wasn't my reality. I am very grounded into the physical manifestation of being here. I have that logical left-brain bias of a trained accountant. I do know I always intuitively conduct my yoga classes, and even I am surprised by where some of them end up. Eventually I had to conclude that they were coming from a part of me that wasn't my logical brain. I have often quipped that my superpower of choice was "intuition", could I go one step further and call those yoga sessions as channelling? Definitely! Especially when I started to receive information that was for my own personal growth as well as my clients.

I was facilitating the first of the 35 Day Detox programs. Initially running them in the familiarity of my studio, and then off-site at the Kāpiti Women's Centre. Of the 13 who initially enrolled for this cycle, 11 were still attending – this had to be my number 1 priority. The triathlon was third on the list and without a second thought it was gone.

* * *

As the internal dialog changes, the external life mimics that change. At a fundamental level the vibrations no longer match. This might be great as you do inner work and wake up without the desire for alcohol or any chocolate ravings. The downside is when friends and family disappear from your life. We often define ourselves by the company we keep. As the journey into self is largely a solitary one it can be hard to stand in that aloneness. It is easy to try to hold relationships that have passed their "use-by" date. And equally easy to grasp hold of the next relationship that matches where you are at. There is also the possibility of meeting people that are in the future, but you have work to do before that connection can fully manifest. This is the minefield of self-understanding and being honest about where you are at.

I have spent numerous hours in recent years contemplating how to raise my own vibration sufficiently that a difficult situation would dissolve out of my life. Sometimes it works. Things do evaporate into a puff of nothingness, other times the situation stays but the emotional response goes.

It was time to add the next piece of the puzzle. The connection to Spirit. At this point I ordered a water filter, for me it was time to take the fluoride out. Discussion abounds in the yoga circles about the calcification of the pineal gland, and how it will hold back spiritual connection. Since my mother had consumed fluoride tablets throughout her pregnancy with me there was a fair chance mine was calcified. The good news was I don't have very many fillings in my teeth. I had none until I was in my mid-thirties.

My beloved Kindle died on the trip to Hawaii and I hadn't replaced it. I tried to find a paperback book worth reading in Waikiki Beach. An almost impossible task! The right book was in the ABC store though – "The Secrets and Practice of Hawaiian Herbal Medicine" by June Gutmanis, the 1976 book had just been re-released. This book gave me further confidence to use the plants in my garden to heal at a deeper level. Thank you.

Conversely once I got to the Ala Moana shopping mall and the Barnes & Noble bookstore, I couldn't find a fiction worth buying that didn't have themes of murder, suspense, and all the other negative vibrations. Maintaining a visual diet of positive images shortened the list of TV shows and movies that I could tolerate too.

Now I was being drawn to YouTube, and not long after that I began listening to the teachings of Kyron. Kyron is a channel by Lee Carrol. In all honesty I cannot tell you exactly what the message was as within a few minutes of starting the video I fell asleep and woke up as it ended. So much so that I eventually gave up checking if it was a recording I had already played and clicked it on anyway. A bit like the Yoga Nidra sleep mediation I had relied on some years earlier. I picked up the concept of "a third language", which spoke to me as to how the vibration behind the message was as important (or perhaps more important), than the practical message itself. This is the case in guided meditations and the resting pose (shavasana) at the end of most yoga classes. Students often worry they will not wake but I have never experienced myself (or others) stay asleep. That type of sleep is the alpha state with 8-13 Hz. You are sub-consciously aware of what is happening.

The penny dropped that success and happiness (in whatever form you define it), will only truly come from within once you are aligned with purpose. To align with purpose means going beyond the gratification of Self (Body and Mind). In 2014 I had argued long and hard that the by-line of the recipe book would be "manifesting change". To me that meant more than wishing for it – it meant being prepared to do the work to align with Soul, to drop what the Mind (ego) wants and find acceptance in everything.

First though it was time to clear karma. A bit like the rocks in the road. All very well to be on the right road, not so good if all you are doing is tripping over the rocks (and sometimes boulders) along the way. It was becoming increasingly obvious to me that each astrological cycle had a lesson in it. By looking at the planetary placements there is a hint as to which part of the life the lesson is. And once it is a lesson it can be approached with the tools in the kitbag. Mostly for me that meant working out how to vibrate my way out of the situation. It also involved a lot of affirmations that I had already overcome the situation. And most importantly that it was cleared from my body's memory.

CHAPTER 33

Queenstown 2018 - Marathon

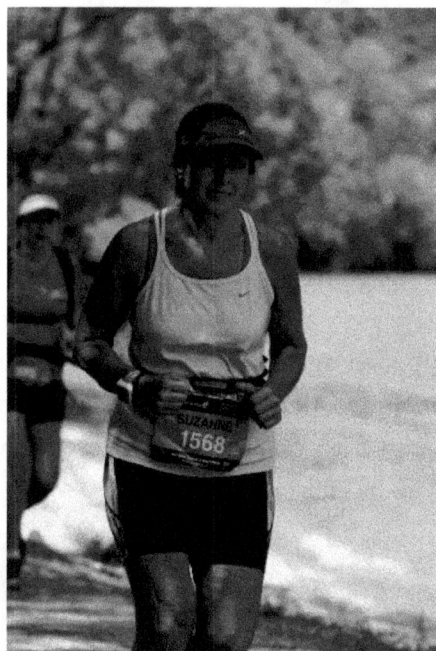

After many years of traveling to Napier and Taupō for events the suggestion was made that we go further afield and run in the Queenstown marathon in the South Island. The Queenstown marathon was part of the Air New Zealand Runaway Marathon Series (in those pre-pandemic days). One of the women had done a Half Marathon there and described it (perhaps incorrectly) as rolling hills. It really appealed to go off-road and be part of the stunning scenery between Arrowtown and Queenstown.

In some bizarre rite of passage – each time I train for a long-distance event there is an almost obligatory fall. In the lead-up to the Taupō Marathon in 2015 I was running around the Dubai Marina. Construction workers had created a mini-wooden bridge to transverse the exposed pipes. On the second 7km loop I didn't lift my foot high enough – and went sprawling on the concrete. Knees and hands cut. This time it was a moment of in-attention as I was running alongside the Kāpiti expressway. Beau was running as "lead dog" (tethered to me at the waist) as two cyclists came towards us. He has a bad habit accessing his farm-dog DNA and wishing to round up cyclists! We went by the first, I looked over my shoulder with relief, and he decided to turn and gather them both. Knees and hands cut again, pride more so as I jumped up to see who had witnessed me going down.

When this happened again a year later, knees and hands cut for a third time, I concluded that it was a potential "bail-out" point. If I wanted a good reason to call time on an event these were all close enough to race day to be legitimate reasons.

* * *

My usual careful arrangements of arriving a day early, and returning a day later were self-sabotaged by a 35 Day Detox Challenge Workshop I had agreed to facilitate. Still it would be good to get away. Ken and I had spent many happy times in Queenstown, I knew the town well, and I thought it would be good for my soul. Hallelujah, this time it was.

Race day was cool and calm. We waited patiently for the bus to take us out to the start line. I relaxed thinking everything was under control. There was a minor panic when I realised that we would only just make it to the start-line in time. I took a deep breath and affirmed that everything was as it should be. We started running slowly. Those first kilometres through Arrowtown were incredible. As the sun heated up, so did the intensity of the hills. Soon we were a bit like mountain goats going up and down single file tracks around Lake Hayes. So much for the rolling hills. Near the river music was playing, it was easy to stay positive. I had plenty of food, but extra water was needed from the aid stations. Major cramps in my calf muscles slowed me down. I was able to continue, there was a long run around the lake front. Beautiful cool air under the trees in the park, and a crowd cheering us on through the township. Throughout the run I sensed Ken's spirit was with me.

Sometimes the lessons we learn are from watching others and being sure that we will do the opposite. Dad had passed when my mother was in her fifties, as was I. What I observed in the next 20 years was shaping the way I approached being widowed. After I had hung up from talking to Mum on that Sunday morning I turned to Ken and screamed at him, "if you ever do that, I'll kill you". Him not at all phased said, "not a problem as I'll already be dead." Bless him for lightening the situation and recognising the shock I was in. But then he went and did it anyway.

At this point I was approaching three years into widowhood. Although I could tick off a few things that I felt I was doing right there was much of the pattern from my mother that I was repeating. Being on your own is difficult. Humans have evolved into a societal structure that requires dependency on others. Some things are very obvious – e.g. few people grow all their own food. Others are not so obvious. On my own

I had to take responsibility for my own wellbeing in the broader sense of the word. I did not have parents to defer to, or children to protect (or defer to). Relationships with friends and extended family change when it is not a "couple" dynamic. Small coping mechanisms crept in that didn't seem much initially, cumulated to make life a smaller version of what it once was. The only exception to that was when I pulled out my passport and got back on a plane. Well, that was true to the extent I never did have an issue with seeing retired couples having the overseas experience together. I was too busy watching it from the self-righteous position of doing something other than a holiday.

The very word "widow" was everything I was fighting so hard against. I did not want this to define me. I wanted this to be a new chapter – one where I stepped into my power and created a new life. I did not want to feel diminished in any way. I wanted to be vulnerable without being dis-empowered. I had to learn not confuse power with control. Control requires tension and effort. Power comes from within and is not stressful.

I had to go beyond the coping strategies, clear the negative energies and seek their positive alternatives. My mantra stopped being about "finding courage" and began to be about "finding joy".

That night I was exhausted and hungry. No way we were walking the kilometre into town. Better get a taxi. The next morning, we woke to a fresh coat of snow throughout the region. How lucky had we been. Time to head back to Kāpiti, finish the program at the Women's Centre and get ready to head overseas.

From my travel journal – December 2018 – Wellington Airport:

"Sri Lanka is calling. After another massive year of personal growth. I am embarking on the next stage of my healing journey. What I have

learnt during the year was that I took on other people's energy – slowing myself down to keep at their pace. Only when I was about to sell the house and downsize did I realise what was happening. After the Queenstown marathon I felt confident to say the job is done and now the pieces can go back together, and I can emerge as the new version of me."

"Transiting through Dubai gave me a sense of what my life used to be like. And I almost think I can recall what my goals were back then."

To become whole, I needed to balance the inner masculine and feminine energies. Having been pushed out of the dependency I thought suddenly everything would be a bed of roses. I was independent. The price of coasting is dependency. I wasn't dependent, but I was coasting. It was a bit like getting in a car for the first time and not being told how to drive. How does this body/mind/soul/spirit physical entity work? Enter the understanding of the masculine and feminine energies at play within us all. The Yin and the Yang. The masculine responsible for the creation and action, the feminine the receptivity and nurturing. One will not work without the other. But what about the distorted versions of both. Out of balance and the distorted masculine will bully and control to get things done. The distorted feminine behaviour will manipulate and beguile to achieve a desired result. These play out in gender roles, though it is important to remember we have both and just like left and right-hand dominant, we can be out of balance in either direction.

This is about going within to identify the patterns. Everything has an outer manifestation that serves to shine a light on what is happening internally. For me, I could sit in that distorted feminine energy of victimhood for a very long time being very frustrated with the lack of progress. Equally I could choose the distorted masculine side and push my way through at the expense of others (and my health) – but I had "been there, done that" (and got the t-shirt to prove it).

My new career had to maintain the principle of authenticity, which for me meant coming back to that place of the true inner masculine energy – particularly the ability to create (manifest). Not just the intuition to find the carpark; but the right people, in the right place, at the right time for my highest good.

In support of this growing awareness my relationship with astrology was changing. Some years earlier I had moved from the Polansky books and started to follow the US astrologer, Susan Miller and her written monthly forecasts. Now it was time to shift again. Following the thread of comments on YouTube I found myself connecting to US Astrologer Molly McChord. Her teachings resonated as they talked of the divine feminine and masculine principles. They introduced me to the Asteroids and evolutionally astrology for soul growth. A bit like how the planets Uranus, Neptune and Pluto were only found as humanity evolved to being in the higher octaves, I believe that these other Asteroids are mimicking developing our collective consciousness.

In 2002 then US Secretary of Defense Donald Rumsfeld explained the limitations of knowledge. His last line stuck in my head - "we don't know what we don't know". It is a great way to humble myself and be open to the possibility that there is more than I realise at play here – things to explore and learn from.

CHAPTER 34

Sri Lanka 2018 - Ayurveda and Yoga Retreat

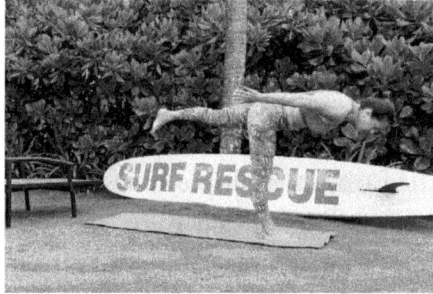

Back to Sri Lanka – no teacher training this time though - it was about nurturing myself. I was done with learning. I had dredged the bottom of the barrel so many times. It was time to put myself back together. My interest in yoga was compelling, but years before that I had been interested in its sister science - Ayurveda.

Ayurveda is India's traditional healing. A bit like TCM (Traditional Chinese Medicine). I had picked up a book on a stopover through

Singapore many years earlier. It was Dr Robert E. Svoboda's 1999 book "AYURVEDA FOR WOMEN a guide to vitality and health". This very tattered copy is still in my collection. Reading this book was perhaps the first time I had understood that we have a "constitution", an inherent tendency towards certain characteristics and traits.

Here is the danger of self-diagnosis though. In 2007 I concluded that I was a "kapha" type and proceeded to implement the healing techniques for that. This is our brain manipulating our perception to keep things as they are. As I bought into the kapha label, I cemented the behaviours that were keeping me stressed. In 2015 I visited a NZ Ayurveda practitioner and she suggested I was Pitta.

* * *

Back in 2011 when I signed up for the YTT I had contemplated going to Sri Lanka to an off-grid retreat. There was no cell phone coverage, no electricity and it sounded like heaven to the stressed executive that I was. I pored over the online brochure for weeks, almost booking, and then closing the browser multiple times. I just could not consider what the response would be if I said I was going into the jungle for a fortnight on my own. While I dithered, the wheels of fate turned, I took the "easy" option of learning to teach yoga in Dubai.

Now randomly that same retreat was in my Facebook news feed. I had not remembered the name – or was I consciously looking for retreats – but there was a sign – it was the answer to the question of how to cope with Christmas on my own. Solution, go away and spend the actual day in the front end of an Emirates plane.

Was I free of obligations now? Not quite. My mother's dementia was progressing at a fast pace. We'd spent the previous Christmas day together as a family, but it was very difficult for everyone, and clear that it would be the last time.

I gave the phone number of the retreat to my sister, there was little more I could do. HelpX visitors came to look after the house and dogs. Time to look after myself.

On arrival in Sri Lanka the hotel transport picked me up and delivered me to the Hotel near Negombo. Two days to decompress with air-conditioning, swimming pool and leisurely breakfast buffets. The first morning I went out for a run along the beach. It felt safe and interesting, but where was the town? I was in no-man's-land, that space close to international airports, where everyone is transiting onwards to somewhere else. It felt like the perfect metaphor for my life.

Soon it was time for the 4-hour drive to Ulpotha. I had learnt from past excursions and arrived with the main group to stay the full two weeks. I didn't have any books to read, notes to take, classes to sequence; and I booked to do all the daily Ayurveda treatments.

When it is described as "off-grid" there is a romantic perception of being at one with nature. And although I love nature, I prefer it to be slightly removed. My version of camping does not stretch to jungle (snakes, spiders, monkeys). I have shared rooms with humans before and didn't mind that. My new definition of security was quickly re-established as the mosquito net, plenty of lavender oil and near constant burning incense to ward off bugs. My daily affirmation had a lot to do with now being immune to mosquitoes. Sadly I did not get past the idea of lurking crocodiles and roaming herds of elephants to explore the local area.

Our first day included a talk from the resident Doctor. Explaining the attributes of the Doshas (life forces/energies) that make up our individual experience. The three main ones being Vata, Pitta and Kapha - plus combinations. According to the doctor I fall into the Pitta/Vata category, which turned out to be the majority of those that check themselves into this retreat.

Based on those Doshas we were each given a list of suggested foods to include/avoid, and a schedule of treatments. The treatments included daily massage, plus periodic saunas, steam baths, oil applications and herbal baths. We practiced yoga twice a day.

Detox symptoms were inevitable – and here I can call myself an expert – so it was interesting to watch it all play out in a traditional and controlled environment. As the days progressed the treatments reached into deeper layers of stored toxins. I experienced some skin rashes (albeit in milder form than I previously had them), but that was about it. Clearly the past seven years of self-experimentation had been effective. I wondered what would have happened if I had arrived in my 2011 state?

Detoxing breaks the attachments. For me astrology supports timing of the spiritual evolution of the physical self. We get the opportunity regularly to cycle round and break another attachment. Some will creep back until the root cause is addressed. Others will go and never return.

* * *

There is a long history of fasting for spiritual growth in many cultures. One I was particularly interested in (from my Middle East days) was the holy month of Ramadan. It occurs during the ninth month of the Muslin calendar. Starting on the new moon and finishing when the next new moon is sighted. Fasting takes place each day between sunrise and sunset. For adults it includes abstaining from food, water, sex, anger, etc. Acts of compassion and kindness are the positive manifestations during this time.

Attachments come in very interesting guises. One recurring theme for many is that of the holidays. The expectations we have written into our psyche about how Christmas, New Year, Mothers/Fathers Day, Birthdays etc "should" be played out. Not only have they been hijacked for commercial gain but they often leave us feeling like we don't measure up in some way. We go to great lengths to fit into our cultural/society's norm. My beliefs around these needed to be shattered. No, it is not "just another day", you can feel there is a special transformational energy that bubbles up around these times. The question is how to reclaim and honour it for its original purpose.

* * *

One afternoon it was time for a group lesson in trust. Time for us to stand in the middle of the circle, close your eyes, turn a few times, and fall, to be caught, be pushed and caught by the others. This time I was comfortable in closing my eyes and surrendering to the moment. Seems I had found trust and tribe within this community.

Having been cocooned in the retreat for the week we had the opportunity to leave the compound and visit a Buddhist temple. The trip into central Sri Lanka had been uneventful – except for the large number of dogs on the roads. It had bothered me a lot about the potential for us hitting one and placed me on high alert. Now that we all piled into the van it should have felt safer. It was a larger group, but the difference was the driver. He thought it a great sport to speed through the villages narrowly missing the animals. By the time we arrived at the temple I was visibly distressed and barely able to speak. Luckily the facilitator saw the problem and I rode in the car with her on the way back.

What it did bring into sharp relief for me was the fact we are prepared to spend our tourist dollars in such a way that condones this behaviour. It is easy to say that there is a problem but, in all consciousness,

I could not contribute to the situation. I made a decision to stop travelling to countries that do not align with my values. Beyond that I now questioned the idea of tourism per se. Was it right to be flocking to these far-flung places, disrupting the environment and societies?

Time to go home; I lasted all of 10 minutes in the Emirates lounge before pouring a glass of champagne, picking up a prawn cocktail and a plate of cheese and crackers. Yup, for the next 30 hours I re-toxed as though my life depended on it. Yet that also served a purpose as it was such a shock to my system that it created its own purge.

And in this moment of desire for a new life I decided it would be a good idea to cut my long hair. My relationship with my hair goes all the way back to childhood when I wanted long hair like my best friend but my mother refused on the grounds that it would be difficult to care for. Yes like many others of my generation I am the result of the trauma of the pudding bowl and home cut. As a Leo I fully embrace that my sense of self is related to my hair - and would honestly prefer to go to the dentist over the hairdresser. I was overjoyed to learn of the connection of our hair to our intuitive abilities. Now I was determined to release it all. First I had to overcome the realisation that this cut would take away the last of my hair that was present when Ken was still alive.

* * *

Returning home from Sri Lanka I began what was the next phase in my growth. The endurance sports had served its purpose and I identified that I needed to expand out to become whole. And that meant facing business as a significant part of my life. I had quipped at 50 that I would be retired. That didn't mean retired from life. It was time to (metaphorically) put the high heels back on and face my Dharma.

I had not been able to fast (in any form) for the last 4 years. My physical, emotional, and mental state was too precarious. There is a need for strength to undertake any period of fasting. On the back of the time away in Sri Lanka I was ready. Not that I knew it. I just woke up on Valentine's Day. It was Beau's birthday, so I took him for a walk on the beach. I realised that I was not having any "Champagne, Roses and Chocolate" moment. I decided to turn it to my advantage and start a Juice Fast. It was also mid-summer, which is a perfect time to assist with a cleanse. I didn't have any pressing commitments. I took the next two weeks off and turned inwards to focus on my physical healing. I revisited the "colonic" cleanse. This time coming from a gentler and less invasive approach, using herbs instead to assist the purging. This option was available at the Ayurvedic retreat, but I rejected the idea of spending money on a holiday – just to sit in the bathroom. From this space of stillness, I began to craft a vision as to what I really wanted for my life going forward.

* * *

Let's talk high heels for a moment. Walking on your toes changes the centre of gravity. Heels tip you forward and put pressure on the hips. Yes, you stand taller, and therefore can feel a sense of empowerment. But that has come at the cost of a less stable base. Externally the perception is that of limitation and vulnerability. The need to be helped in some way. Physically they shorten the calf muscles and lock the ankles. At worst they deform the foot, forcing toes to curl back on themselves.

One yoga teacher friend correctly refers to all shoes as foot coffins. Not only do we lose connection with the Earth, but we lose the stabilizing muscles of the foot, forcing the knees and hips to bear that load. Not what those major joints are designed for. But like many of us, I was prepared to sabotage myself in many random ways for some perceived benefit of fitting in.

One of my favourite internal dialogues is "Just because you can doesn't mean you should." This gives me the ability to acknowledge the mind's input but gently override those thoughts for a greater good. Works equally for food choices, reluctance to go out for a training run, or hesitation to move forward in life itself.

CHAPTER 35

Wellington 2019 - Half Marathon (take 3)

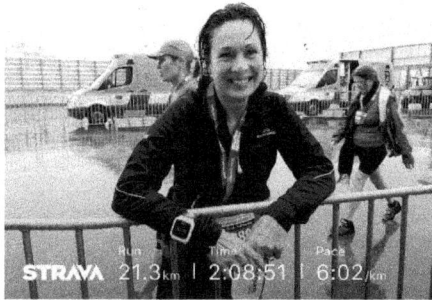

STRAVA 21.3km | 2:08:51 | 6:02/km

Driving in early – ridiculously early – I felt very alone. This was not how I saw my life playing out. I'd returned from Sri Lanka with a belief that the grieving process was over, and I was consciously choosing "joy". I may have been running faster than ever before but the outer manifestation wasn't matching the inner desire for happiness.

My question was "how to trust that there will be a positive outcome when so much had gone wrong?" Burying the past was no longer an option, it had to come up, be acknowledged, only then it could be released. When we envisage an outcome, it is tainted by our experience of what has previously happened. Either to ourselves, our family, or perhaps history itself. It cements a repeating cycle and robs us of the opportunity to grow.

By now I knew that just because a lesson was learnt it doesn't mean it will not come back. My experience is that it comes back again at another level. A little like the university curriculum that has a 101, 201, and 301 course structure.

I needed to find the things that were going right and only focus on those. I decided to release my expectations on the outcomes of everything else. To conquer this, I approached the race with the intent of running as I had never done before. I knew that I was physically capable of the run. I acknowledged the power of my mind to remain focused and positive. And I dropped all expectations of an outcome. I said to myself I would run this race as if my future life depended on it.

* * *

A few months earlier, on the morning of my mother's funeral I realised that I wasn't in a fit state to drive into Wellington. Although she had been ill for as long as Ken, I didn't appreciate the impact her passing would have. I'd learnt something over the years and this time I was willing to ask for help. A quick call to the funeral celebrant and I was picked up and driven into Wellington. Sitting by myself in the chapel was excruciating as all the family resentments and dysfunction were played out. A photo of Mum, Dad and Ken together was displayed. That was the point of understanding that the three closest people to me were now all gone. I was no longer a wife or a daughter.

Society has expectations of us. Mostly in the form of the word "should". One of Ken's rhyming sayings came back to me "should've, would've, could've, didn't". He did not conform to anyone else's expectations. He was the polar opposite to me who conformed before it was even an expectation. Deeply reflecting on my life, I could sense that I wasn't free. And yet it seemed from the outside looking in that I would be.

What was holding me back? Parasites. In one of those moments of insight I saw that part of my ongoing battle with sugar was related to gut issues and issues for the second chakra (again). Bingo, I was probably feeding the parasites. A quick explanation of parasites is "organisms that feed off the host". Physically they are found on the skin, in the mouth, and in the gut.

Taking an approach that everything reflects everything else, I asked these questions of myself.

- Where was I dependent on others?
- Where were others dependent on me?
- How would that be manifesting in the physical body?

I was on to something – and it was time to look for foods that would be feeding the parasites. Namely my old nemesis – sugar.

Sugar is not just the white stuff that is as addictive as cocaine. It is the fruit sugars, honey, and syrups. Training was burning them fast as fuel but that didn't mean it was healthy. I often would say I would rather feel physically sick from overeating than to feel the emotions behind a situation. For me that is emotional eating – not so much eating to feel better – rather eating to not feel. Keeping the second chakra blocked by overloading the digestive system.

And it's not just what we eat but how we eat too. It's easy to eat while on the move, or while watching TV, or scrolling an electronic device. There is no point having the healthiest salad and serving it with a side of anger, frustration, or loneliness.

Time and again there is a kickback. We initiate change and make progress and then the Universe comes along with a test to see if we were serious about the change. Sometimes we pass, sometimes we fail. After taking action I felt better and my gut health was massively improved. A lot of the bloating was gone and the redness in my skin started to dissipate. That was funny, as I looked in the mirror and realised that my ears didn't need to be red!

Better still, I had found a use for Ken's Bombay Sapphire Gin. It was one of the ingredients in a scrub that helped clear my Rosacea and Psoriasis. Both of which can be associated with an element of parasitic infection.

* * *

I signed up to do IronMāori 2019 – not because I particularly wanted to do it. More that some of the other women would be there – and I felt like I was adrift – needing an event to pull me back into "normality".

Usually I would be into training by the last week of August – or first week of September. This year that wasn't the case. I was busy being busy with work and some personal issues were hanging heavily on me. Four weeks out and I hadn't been on my bike yet. And then it happened – I tripped in a moment of in-attention while running with Beau. Not his fault but because we were tethered, he pulled me along in the gravel. I probably needed stitches on my knees but by the time I had got home (washing the gravel out in the sea), I found some old suture tape, and put myself back together. Now I had ensured there was no way I would be in Napier. In many ways I was relieved.

After the DNF in Kinloch at the beginning of 2018 I was following up with a DNS for Napier at the end of 2019. Sometimes we pass a test, sometimes we fail.

Out the window went the healthy eating. I was fuelling on way too many sugars. Soon my heels started to crack and I was developing a yeast infection on my upper back. It was like watching a train wreck in slow motion. Often I would unfollow people on the training app Strava as I could see their overtraining leading to injury, missed events and disappointment. I was doing exactly the same thing; except I wasn't doing the overtraining bit – just the train wreck impersonation.

Tests only come from the Universe around something that is important. If it didn't have an personal emotional blueprint it wouldn't qualify as a test.

By now I knew the pattern of being tested; two steps forward, and one step back. Napier IronMāori wasn't the only event I had signed up for earlier in the year. Let's say I must have been hedging my bets because I had also booked accommodation for the Queenstown Marathon (six weeks away) and entry to the Taupō Half Ironman (in eight weeks' time).

* * *

Could I pull myself out of the current downward spiral and commit to achieving something at the tail-end of 2019? There was a new moon coming and I could catch that energy. More importantly though was the buzz in astrology community of the Solar Eclipse on Boxing Day and Pluto Saturn conjunction in January. David Palmer, The Leo King Astrologer was describing this period (November) of being onboard with doing the inner work - or missing the proverbial boat. Not something I was keen to do. I didn't come this far to give up now!

My goals for the coming cycle were:

- Home - create a safe and nurturing environment.
- Relationships - choose the high vibes of joy, love and companionship.
- Finances - ensure revenue exceeds expenditure.
- Personal - parasites be gone!

CHAPTER 36

Taupō 2019 - Half Ironman (take 3)

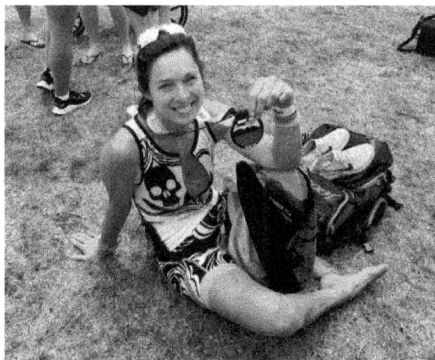

This was make or break time for me and triathlon. I had done this event in 2014 and 2016 and would say they were both my favourite events. I thought I would either be enthused to buy a new bike and get back into triathlon or I would sell my hot pink Avanti.

I did lots of running. Very little swimming (once a week max) and continued to do yoga with my clients. What I didn't do was hills on the bike. By now I was riding solo and had lost my confidence to venture beyond the city limits.

My biggest interest was in strength training. Each week I was in the gym doing weight training. I felt strong. A friend had encouraged me to join her at the gym. It wasn't a scientific approach, but it worked for me. We started at the first machine and worked our way along them all. She was very practical and read the instructions and then we backed each other to give it a try. Initially we used no weights and completed only one or two sets. After a few weeks, we increased the weights, and we were doing three sets of each. This was a challenge I could really get behind because it was measurable – and fun.

At the Half Ironman event, the swim was the first time I had not resorted to backstroke. The strength training had helped, but so too had the mental strength and calmness of mind. The lake was calm, and the water was warm. It was a pleasure and privilege to be there. The bike was harder than I remembered but it felt good. There was only wind on the return – and all I could think of was that at least I didn't have to go around and do the 90kms again. No bike mechanical issues and I just had the 21kms to run. Now this was my strong point. For the last two years I had mostly run. I was in a good place to "put to rest" the trauma of the Ironman run.

Not so, within 3kms (on the first rise) both quads cramped on me. Not a minor pain but a "stop you dead in your tracks" level of pain. My legs couldn't move. I had to stop. I couldn't even walk. When have I not been able to walk in a race?

Other participants stopped and asked if I was okay. Did I need a medic? I didn't know. I stood and held a lamppost for a while and thought perhaps I could hobble to the aid station and get help. I didn't have any support people with me. I was on my own. From the back of my mind came the story from the KWT Coach - that the mind can only focus on one source of pain at a time. Ken's version was a little more gruesome – and includes stories of sailors chopping a thumb off to distract the patient having a leg amputated. What if I gave my mind something else to think about? Would the cramp release? I picked up sharp pebbles and jammed them into the palms of my hands. I could now move - forward to the aid station that was within sight.

I explained the problem of the cramps and asked for advice. Their suggestion was a gel and perhaps some ice. I took both and threw the ice down my front and back. Swapping the pebbles for ice I clutched cubes in my hands and started to walk to the next station. I had nothing to prove. I could walk off the course and be done with all this drama. Why was I still here? It was the answer I was looking for. I didn't need to do this anymore. As I walked I justified quitting when I got back to the transition area. There was no way I was doing two more laps. I crossed paths with one of my Kāpiti buddies. Maybe I could just run a few steps to at least show some effort.

The battle between my body and mind was real. I was in pain, something that hadn't been the case on the 2017 Taupō Ironman run. Was I doing permanent damage? Or was it temporary? Eventually I was able to run periodically. And continue walking with the ice in my hands. Forward to the finish line. After all that drama I was still within the time of my previous race in 2016. What did I think? I may even be able to get in under 7 hours.

Here's my social media post:

"Done and it included a sprint finish. I looked at my watch and it was 6 hrs 41 mins. Of course I would think I wonder if I can get under 7 hrs - 6:59:23. I am the ultimate "just made it" artist.

Feet up with cramps from the hills on the bike and trying to run them back to relaxed. Under 40 mins for the swim - amazing result right there.

Not a perfect day but very happy with myself."

For the first time I crossed the finish line with a smile on my face and my hands in the air – why - because I knew that I would never do this again. Truly within the next couple of months all the triathlon kit was on Trademe. I was strong physically and mentally. I had faced the pain and not hurt myself or sold myself short. I had run myself to empty and come away happy. I had learnt all that I could from endurance racing.

* * *

Years later I was researching the impact of the asteroid "Chiron" on a person's birth chart. Chiron is referred to as the "wounded healer". It represents the part of your life where you have spiritual work to do. Chiron entered in the sign of Pisces in 2011 and crossed my natal position (4 degrees 53 minutes) in mid-February 2012. The Chiron Return happens once in a lifetime (approximately 50 years) and brings up everything that has not yet been healed. In effect it is the reset button as you now go back to the beginning – this time armed with the wisdom of the first half of life. This was my true healing crisis – sitting in my seventh house of relationships (focus on partnerships in all areas of my life, including the higher self). Chiron left Pisces in 2019. I was right when I called it that day, I had learnt all I could about the body and mind and spirit as it relates to the physical manifestation of self.

* * *

It was time to learn about coming back to life. Continually focusing on what was wrong was not helping me to live a better life. I might have become very good at clearing karma and working my way through those blocks but it didn't have a positive energetic vibration. A "better life" could only come from a "happier" life.

I began to understand the true meaning behind the 35 Day Detox by-line "manifesting change". It was necessary to step beyond where I was at and move into what I wanted. But what did I want? It was not clear. So much of my efforts had been about what I didn't want. And the tangible "things" that had been priorities before, no longer had any interest.

The book "The Law of Attraction" outlines the way in which our positive thoughts bring in the heart's desire. Great if you want to focus on that new car, house, job, or holiday. Not helpful if you cannot find something that you want sufficiently to stimulate an emotional response. Because without the emotion behind the desire, the law of attraction does not work.

As I came out of the fear response, I was able to move beyond the point of focusing on everyday survival needs and this created an opportunity for reflection as to what is truly important. It can also activate an "existential crisis". This is deeper than depression and anxiety, yet it can be wrapped up in the same packaging. This made total sense to me as I ticked a lot of the influencing factors:

- A history of repressed emotions
- Loss of a loved one
- Guilt
- Feeling socially unfulfilled
- Dissatisfied with self

The layer upon layer of guilt we wear is such a complex subject. We feel guilty for so many things – and it holds us back from enjoying life. Eventually it leads back to the guilt you feel within yourself for not meeting your own expectations. Drop any expectations you have of yourself, and you can drop the guilt.

I needed to clear the emotions I couldn't see but knew were there. The opportunity to engage in therapy presented itself. Not once but multiple times it was in my face. I was in the garden feeling sorry for myself and one therapist literally stopped the car and suggested I call her. My reluctance was born of a belief that talking about the problem wouldn't solve the problem. It would allow me to co-exist with the problem, but it would not clear it. I had no interest in living in this space as (apart from the responsibility for my two dogs) I had nothing to keep me tethered here.

Enter sound vibration therapy!

Initially I was drawn to the healing frequencies of the chakras. Soon I was listening to some of the chants from my yoga teacher trainings. The sounds of the chants have healing properties. When we take it one step further, we can surmise that some of our spoken words do have a negative vibration. Not just in their meaning – but in the frequencies themselves. As we take negative words and normalise them into everyday use we absorb and lower the bar (our frequency), i.e. listening to yogis swearing is an antithesis of what living a yogic lifestyle is.

Researching sound vibration brought me to the Solfeggio frequencies. The premise that all the organs of the body have a unique frequency. If the organ is healthy, it will be in harmony with a sound wave of the same frequency. If it is out of balance the sound can help with recalibration. It explained the fact that although I love being by the beach - I cannot stand the sound of the waves. Surprise, surprise the frequency of the Ocean matches to the Heart Chakra. As I started to connect with the various frequencies, the emotional reaction was immediate and profound. My meditation practice was now a daily deep-dive into the YouTube channel of Meditative Mind. This free resource is phenomenal; I know the effect it has had on my life; reading the comments suggest that this is true for thousands of others around the globe too.

Incorporating a bit of tough love, I concluded the frequencies that annoyed me the most were probably the ones I needed to listen to. Very soon I found myself back with the yoga chants of Ganesha (remover of obstacles), the Gayatri Mantra (being open to learning) Moh Mohiya (letting go), and Ajai Alai (finding inner power). Listening each morning to a random chant on the Meditative Mind channel of YouTube was profoundly healing. It created an emotional outpouring, followed by a subsequent feeling of peace.

The internal conflict about not caring for my mother in her final years took centre stage. I was asking myself:

- What does it mean to "live a good life"?
- When do we cut ourselves a break that we cannot live up to others' expectations?
- When do we choose ourselves as a priority?

All this conditioning needs to go to find peace from within. Once the peace is internal, the external environment will follow suit and life becomes more serene.

I watched Jojo (Mum's dog) morph from an uncontrollable nuisance; one that needed to be muzzled to walk her on the beach, to a dog that was friendly (with the occasional outburst), and finally to a placid likable dog that was referred to as "adorable". Was she the same dog? I may have done some cord-cutting between her, Mum and I and placed a very large Obsidian crystal in her bed. Obsidian is said to block psychic attacks and absorb negative energies.

What was really changing was my energy. I was acknowledging that my mother's behaviour was coming from an unconscious place. She had chosen a very difficult soul contract for this incarnation. The ultimatum she had issued in 2015 was only another trigger for my personal growth.

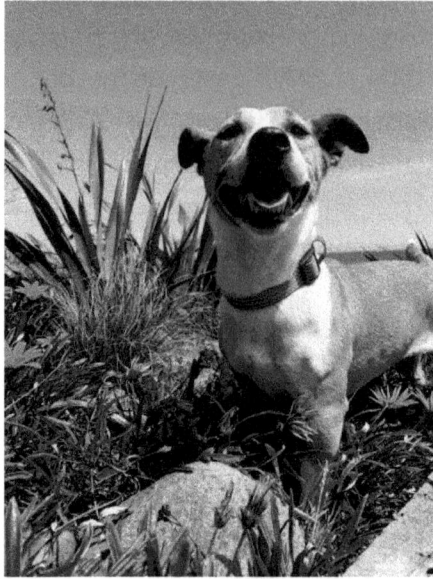

There is a part of me that would like to honour my mother with a tattoo – as I did with Ken. Yet those wounds run even deeper. If it happens it will be the starfish. On the Kāpiti Coast I seldom see them on the beach. On her passing there was the largest one washed up on to the shore. I looked up the symbolism and "they have the ability to lose a limb and continue". Now I periodically see them on the shore, and I always realise that the issue at hand may cause the loss of something, but I will always recover, and grow from the experience.

So, although I had lost much in the last five years, I had equally grown to the point where I could say she was my greatest teacher.

CHAPTER 37

Lockdown 2020

My first thought as the yoga studio closed was – well I will finally write "that" book (spoiler alert, it didn't happen). The criticism of the 2014 recipe book "35 Day Detox – Manifesting Change" was that it didn't have my story in it. That was valid. At the time I was in no place to add a personal narrative. Besides, the book was originally written with the intention of being my private record of healthy and healing recipes.

In January 2020 I had co-hosted a workshop on personal planning for 2020. Even with all the practical business skills and esoteric skills the co-host and I imparted that day, I could not see how my year was going to unfold. Everything I had initiated was floundering. Unseen forces stopped me from going where I thought I "should" be, e.g. opening a new yoga/wellbeing space, doing retreats and workshops, hosting Airbnb wellness clients.

* * *

As I deepened my meditation practice it appeared as if my life was falling apart. I know the connection between the inner world and the outer manifestation of the home environment. It's one of the core principles of the 35 Day Detox; a way to hack the transformation process! And just when I thought I couldn't deal with anything else in my life, a series of seemingly random events occurred.

The kitchen taps broke, the dishwasher blocked, the lights short circuited, the air-conditioning unit seized, and my personal favourite – a low battery on the security system set off the house alarm one evening. The sirens screamed throughout the house and in sheer desperation I found the garden secateurs and cut the wires.

My life was being re-arranged before my very eyes. At least now I understood this to be the case and could find the positive viewpoint.

* * *

Was it locked down or locked up?

All thoughts of yoga went out the window and my personal and professional practice disappeared.

On the day New Zealand went into the first lockdown a friend visited, their last words were that they would check in soon. I knew I would be doing this without any support of family. I shut the gates and went to lie on the bed. I closed my eyes and it all came rushing back. I was back in Dubai on that fateful day in February 2012.

The call came through the fog from the prison warden – "Mrs Stokes". I'm not sure I even heard it. I was nudged awake by the Indonesian lady. "That's you isn't it?". I made my way to the door and was asked to follow one of the prison guards.

I was used to walking corridors like this. However, I was always dressed in appropriate business suits with high heels. The trick was to walk fast enough to keep up without making this ridiculously loud noise that echoed down the hall. Now I had flat shoes on, maybe I was imagining it, but everyone was looking. Perhaps it was because I was one of the few westerners here, or maybe my age, or the clearly expensive clothes. At the best of times I prefer to stay in the background, but there was no hiding this walk of shame. Inside the office was the Colonel, Ken, and an Egyptian Lawyer.

They agreed that no money was outstanding, but until an official release was provided by the free trade zone officials there was nothing that could be done. Was I to stay in prison while Ken and the lawyer sorted it out? I was the only one who knew the organisation and how to get through the local system to get the appropriate signatures. Ken would have deferred it to me – but I wasn't in any position to help. And yet I was the one suffering here. Eventually a potential solution was tabled. If Ken handed over his passport, I could be released to sort out the administration over the next 72 hours. At least I wouldn't be spending the night in prison.

I would like to have thought that there was no debate about this. It was the obvious win-win for everyone. Except that Ken was reluctant to let go of his passport. Without it he couldn't leave the country. Under my breath I said, "Why would you want to leave the country when your wife is in prison." To make matters worse this was not even a company that I had any business interest in. Back in 2010 I had been doing Ken a favour by arranging the lease! His failed business acquisition – that ensured I couldn't continue my corporate career - had come back and bitten us hard.

We returned to the hotel at midnight with the lawyer who explained to Reception my lack of passport – and the letter that I had in its place.

I didn't make eye contact with anyone or say a word. We closed the door to the room and only then did I start to shake uncontrollably.

* * *

I'm not sure where the line is between courage and stupidity. Since you have got this far on my journey through this book, you know that I did return to Dubai on several occasions. What may have looked like a chilled time mixing a bit of work, holiday and yoga teacher training was a very real battle to control my fear. Each visit through Dubai Airport Terminal 3 was my Armageddon. The sights, the sounds, the smells, all triggered a deep visceral fear response.

Locked up at home in New Zealand should have been easy. I had everything I needed, and we were enjoying a late summer. There was access to the amazing beach, and over 1,500 acres of Queen Elizabeth Park. I had clients on the 35 Day Detox Program and in the Facebook support group but they were in the same state of shock and there was little to divert my attention there. The use of social media to create virtual connections initially seemed a great way to go. Ultimately though, it became a distraction from what was really happening. There was more personal healing work to be done – and that's not possible while engaged and distracted.

* * *

For me it's interesting to look behind my messages on social media and see where I have a need for validation, connection, or relevancy. We construct lives that look important and busy on the outside but many of the activities are other people's idea of fulfilment. I was buying into that storyline.

During those weeks did I even run? No, I was paralysed with fear again. Where was the fear coming from? Much was externally created and easy to switch off. Yet there was something else for me. When you venture out feeling unsafe it is interesting how the mind plays tricks with you. Are the clothes suitable to keep you from being singled out for unwanted attention? Will the car break down and leave you stranded without a way to get home? Do you wear flat shoes in case you need to get home on foot? These are the type of thoughts that surface when you are "going it alone" and highlight how we can quickly undermine a positive mindset.

Beyond this was a deeper issue I had – that of abandonment. Very soon I realised this was the underlying stress response driving my fears. Originating in the first chakra the feelings of abandonment had been triggered, ready for a deeper level of healing.

The answer is to recover the connection between the mind and body. To strengthen the trust that my body is an ally. Daily movement with awareness is key. For me that is yoga – the very thing that flew out the door first. As I say, we don't always pass the test the first time, or even the second. I back myself that it will eventually be "third time a charm" though. Furthermore, I learned that just because I am currently failing a test does NOT mean I am a failure.

At the end of the lockdown, when I thought there was no hope of any international travellers arriving via HelpX, I received a message from a beautiful Chinese soul. She arrived, settled me, and stayed – until it became apparent that others were coming and going, and she was still with me. It was time for her to move on too. Angels come in all forms.

Our animals are also angels sent to help, and a good barometer of what is happening internally. As I watched them act out, I knew that I needed to clear this too – at least for their sake - if not mine.

But it wasn't karma from my actions. Where did it come from? A soul contract between Ken and me? A past life? I couldn't name its source, but I could identify where I was holding it in my body. My upper back was covered with Tinea Versicolor – a yeast infection which started on the corner of the tattoo. "Stabbed in the back?" would be a very good guess. And in a past life, I was probably the one doing the stabbing. If I needed further confirmation at home the boundary fence in the Feng Shui "relationship zone" was demolished leaving me with a very uncomfortable level of exposure and vulnerability.

* * *

When we were locked down for a second time in 2020 things got very interesting. An acquaintance shared a story on social media about sexual abuse in all its different forms. It relates to the second chakra and can be a cause of reproductive and digestive issues, a pattern of shutting down feelings. I didn't give it much attention as my thoughts were elsewhere.

Having cleared so much of my personal baggage I was questioning why I was still alone. It was not something I thought would happen. Ken had said I would find someone else, I thought so too. But did I really want to fall back into that dynamic? I was pretty sure I didn't. Looking back I could see how I had compromised so much of myself to maintain the relationship. I had done that willingly, and at the expense of all other relationships (including the relationship with Self). Was it a lack of self esteem, or self worth? I didn't think so.

Which led me to question why I had a distorted view of intimate relationships. A pattern that had been present throughout my life. Until the morning I was in the garden turning the compost bins – thinking that it was a great metaphor for my life. Just moving the piles around and getting nowhere. Working my way back through all my relationships. Mostly they had all started in the workplace. Finally unpacking the story of getting into trouble as a teenager for lying to my father about going to the movies with a group of friends. We all know the story – boys and cars were involved. He had taken the belt to me – stuff I had uncovered and dealt with – thanks to Dr Phil's Self Matters book. I could verbalise that story without any emotional attachment.

What I had blocked was the inappropriate relationship with the older guy next door. The story I had told no one about; not my parents, not Ken, most importantly not myself. His name was Beau.

I looked at my beautiful boy Beau and just cried. I cried for that younger self who didn't understand a true expression of love and intimacy. All those years of carrying that baggage was too much.

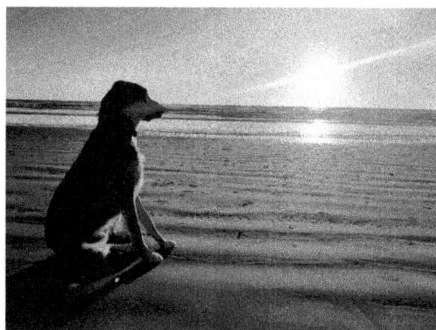

I needed to work through forgiveness to release the trauma from my body, particularly the second (sacral) chakra. My Beau carries the masculine template, and he became the key to healing. He was always the true expression of love (my valentine's puppy), and as he grew up, he became my protector too.

In many ways it is easier to maintain the status quo. This desire to turn inward and face the unpleasant stories is not for the fainthearted. It would have been OK to keep the protective walls up and engage with life through that shield. My feeling though was that would be a disservice and a little like eating sugar-free chocolate or non-dairy cheese. Why bother?

CHAPTER 38

Reflections

What did happen on that first 10km run in Dubai in 2011? I naively thought it was about achieving something physical. Namely the ability to put time aside, invest in myself, and achieve a goal that was purely personal in nature. Or maybe just to have bragging rights that I had done something interesting that Christmas.

Even though it was outside my comfort-zone I had showed up, put one foot in front of the other, and continued until the run was finished. It had plunged me into a world of pain, self-doubt, and self-loathing. As I ran that day, I dredged up a lot of things that I did not like.

Those issues could be summed up as me being a victim of circumstances and people. That I was a failure and wasting a perfectly good life. They came from a feeling of being dis-empowered. Did I want that to be my view of myself? Absolutely not!

The catch cry for the next decade became "something has to change". A softly spoken, but insistent inner voice replying whenever I thought "this is not the day to change", reminding me that actually "maybe this is exactly the day to make a change."

* * *

All this self-reflection was taking me deeper and deeper. I was way past the issues of my childhood and yet the same stories of fear, betrayal and abandonment hovered in the background. Where was this coming from? They ran straight down the matriarchal line.

Both my mother and grandmother had issues with their kidneys. Kidney stones in the first instance, and the removal of a failed kidney in the second. And even though I had chosen to ignore my own prior diagnosis of early signs of kidney disease I carried the cellular memory of their traumas. My physical health was deteriorating despite the healthy diet and regular yoga practice. Was this the ancestral healing coming up to be cleared? Or did I really have a medical problem?

As those changes unfolded life got even trickier. Instead of holding things together I was pushed out of control and at the mercy of what I like to call "the washing machine of life". Tossed around and floundering.

This was when I added the Universe to my list of things I didn't like. I became a victim of that too. Now I was railing against everything. When there is no hope there is only faith. Cue the eighth limb of yoga.

Those eight limbs are:

- Yama – the restraints (or moral code) of behaviour
- Niyama – the healthy habits to maintain
- Asana – the practice of the physical postures
- Pranayama – engaging in breathing techniques
- Pratyahara – withdrawal of the five physical senses (sight, taste, touch, hearing, smell)
- Dharana – control of the mind via concentration

- Dhyana – meditation
- Samadhi – surrender

In those early days of the first YTT we were told that there are two paths to spiritual growth. The first requires the discipline to follow the first seven steps (limbs). The second is where you skip ahead to the eighth limb – Samadhi (surrender). It comes when you stop trying to control life and let it unfold. In effect enter the Universal flow and are guided in all that you do. Surrender refers to trusting in the unseen forces. Those we can't see or prove – except like gravity – by their results or consequences.

Walking the beach each morning I was now repeating this mantra "dear higher self, you are in charge, please guide me to see the right things, do the right things, say the right things, hear the right things, meet the right people." Followed by "dear conscious mind, sub conscious mind and unconscious mind; you heard the message, higher self, she's in charge so relax and let her get on with it!"

That sounds very serene and yogi-like. Often it was more like me stomping up the beach issuing threats and challenges. By the time I turned and returned for the homeward walk things had calmed. Until one of the dogs kicked off at something and I knew I still had a long way to go.

That Universal flow is a little like the school system – at the end of term there will be a test. And tests only come in the areas that are important. If it was something without an emotional attachment it would be easy. But no, tests appear in a particular area of life (and at the exact time) you would rather things stay exactly as it is. That is why they are a test!

How do we know if there is an emotional attachment? Because there is a reaction. For example: The opposite of love is not hate. Hate is an emotion and means that you care. The opposite of love is dis-interest. When there is nothing. When we have disconnected and feel nothing for a person or situation. I like to use "cord-cutting" as a tool to energetically cut the attachments when I've identified them. Taking time to cut, then send healing energy to both parties. It takes two to tango after all. Another tool is this simple mantra:

"I apologise for the pain I have caused you in the past. I forgive you for the pain you are causing me now. The past is past – it's over. Thank you."

* * *

What I hadn't comprehended was the amount of resilience that is needed to grow spiritually, i.e. the ability to withstand a situation, adapt to the circumstances and then to recover from the event (adverse or favourable). I had bucketloads of the former when it came to business endeavours, facing financial hardship, maintaining relationships, and living with health issues. What was missing was the second part of the equation – the ability to adapt. I simply did not see that as an option.

As I sat on the stairs at home one afternoon, I was back in that story of trying so hard and nothing succeeding. The phone rang. I wanted to ignore it. Instead I stood up, raised my arms overhead, took a couple of deep breaths, (the old feeling of panic of potentially missing a call, or receiving bad news, was long gone), and said "Hi". It was an offer of the opportunity to become president of a local networking group for the next six months. As we talked, I walked around the house and, fidgeting with a pot plant, I saw the first shoot of a new flower on the orchid. There were the unseen forces at work. I said yes, who knew where it would lead next?

* * *

If I was to summarise this spiritual growth, I'd say it was all in the numbers! Astrology shows where the story was playing out, the cycles beginning and ending, and what the lessons were. Numerology gave the framework of my journey.

A quick look into the practice of Numerology (and my Personal Year Number) and here is everything that I have experienced in the past 10 years. Could it have been foretold and avoided? No, I believe the universe doesn't work like that. We can see the potential of a situation unfolding however we always have free will as to how we will respond. That is the element of choice. Did I have to keep facing my shadow side and actively work to clear it out of my system? Definitely not, I see a number of choice points where I could have progressed at a more comfortable pace. Not necessarily settling per se – more a case of slowing the pace of change down.

If I hadn't been constantly working the 35 Day Detox Challenge puzzle with clients, it is likely that would have been my story. I advise clients they really can only do a maximum of three cycles before needing to take a breather and let their changing external reality catch up. Often, I would start superficially, going through the motions but once that awareness of a limit is seen it's hard to ignore.

For example, the inexplicable pain in the left elbow.

- Is it tennis elbow? No, in the wrong place,
- OK, then its golfer's elbow.
- By why a pain in the elbow? – energetically representing where we are not embracing life.
- Where am I holding back on enjoying life?
- What is the food that is represented here?
- Is there something I can eat to support the healing?
- How does it show up on the yoga mat?

- Is it time to nurture rather push forward?
- What is my new mantra to tell my body I am healed from the situation?

I heard a description by the US Tarot reader Ericka Elmuts that this personal growth is "like a marathon that you don't know what the distance is". That resonated with me. All my races have had a major element of knowing what the distance is and breaking it down to just make it to the end. What if you needed to get up each day and go again? Like those endurance athletes who do the multi-day ultra-distance events. It requires a different strategy. Not one of working out how much fuel was needed for a single activity, but one where the physical system was so complete in the nourishment of self that showing up (putting one for foot in front of the other) was the natural state of being.

In 2011 I entered a 9 year (the number 9 symbolises endings). A quirk of the system is that the year really doesn't start until your birthday that year. The story line clicks over on January 1st and there is a glimpse of what is coming, and then another glance in April as we start the astrological new year; but the energy changes for me at my birthday in mid-August. All the significant changes in my life occur around this time. So much so that I now schedule a 4-week break then to let life recalibrate.

So here is the decade summarised:

- 2011/12 – year 9 and the end of my corporate life and time in Dubai. The old cycle crashed and burnt with such force that there was nothing to return to.
- 2012/13 – year 1 ushered in beginnings and new directions. Physical activity took centre stage and business became a secondary consideration. As I tried to hold onto the past I had to deal with loss of corporate identity.

- 2013/14 – year 2 was a choice point. Would I embrace the yogic path and become a better version of myself, or would I fall into line with family expectations?
- 2014/15 – year 3 is the commitment to that choice. I doubled down on the healthy lifestyle and threw myself into the writing of the recipe book.
- 2015/16 – year 4 expands and grows those choices. I began to teach the principles of the 35 Day Detox. I matured as I learnt to prioritise my needs first.
- 2016/17 – year 5 brings into the physical realm the change that has been manifesting behind the scenes. Even though I could see it coming and thought I was prepared, I had no idea the depth of what was about to unfold.
- 2017/18 – year 6 restores balance and harmony. After the shock of Ken and Buster's passing, there was a period of settling and regrouping. The old company was finally liquidated.
- 2018/19 – year 7 deepens the spiritual connection. It is the bliss of understanding, or the lesson of reaching for the lifeline when it is thrown. This was when Mum passed and triggered even more growth.
- 2019/20 – year 8 is the manifestation. You reap what you sow. Which is great if you've put the work in, not so if you have missed class too many times. I give myself a "scraped through by the skin of my teeth" result.
- 2020/2021 – year 9 completes the cycle and clears out the old ready for the next cycle to come in.

Much as I would have liked this learning journey to have been over many times through the decade it really didn't shift until 15/8/2021. The day of my 60th birthday. In contrast to 10 years previous when I had been fixated on having a boat party and material possessions, that year I had an appreciation of the ability to connect to the natural environment. In the weeks leading up to the day I began to question whether I had "missed the boat". This is classically referred to as "the dark night of the soul". I felt I had come close but not been able to step through the portal. At the eleventh hour a friend cancelled our plan to have dinner together. I momentarily froze as I wondered if I would be able to endure the weekend on my own. Did I have everything I needed within this version of me?

I did! I walked 4kms down the beach to Paekākāriki with the dogs, we left before dawn and as we returned, I watch a beautiful crisp mid-winter sunrise. I enjoyed preparing delicious food for myself from the recipe book. Then I picked up a brush and started painting the yoga studio.

CHAPTER 39

Lockdown 2021

Two days after my 60th birthday we went back into lockdown in New Zealand. The only two other social gatherings I had planned were also cancelled. This time I thought I was prepared for the shock of change. Truth is you are never prepared for the reality of radical change. By its nature it is something your conscious mind can't see. It takes courage to maintain equilibrium in uncertain times, and all change is inherently uncertain. Even if you know what is happening on a physical level you cannot know how you will react at an emotional level.

I was thrown another lifeline by one of my clients and soon established myself in a daily routine of videoing my personal yoga sessions for YouTube. The real benefit of this exercise came with the analysis afterwards of why I was doing certain poses on those days. Within that reflection I connected to the issues I was currently addressing.

Mostly it came to the point it was time to do life my way. It was time to overhaul my life at a deeper level. To be true to what is important, recognise what is not, and have the courage to walk away where necessary.

Over the past few years, I have often had a kingfisher bird sitting on the fence – he comes at times of indecision and difficult choices to be made. And for me he represents the "giving up of something of value in order to receive something more". He was sitting on the fence looking at me. It was time to take a deep breath and change some fundamental priorities. I frequently teach with the question "are you working to live or living to work" statement. Perhaps I could heed my own advice.

* * *

In 2015 in the YTT we were all tasked with creating class sequences. They were based on Vinyasa principles – and generally had a theme, or a "peak" pose that the class was working towards. I glibly said I didn't plan classes; they came from an intuitive space where I followed the flow of energy. I also have an excellent memory which serves as a fallback position. If I could relax and get into the flow, I knew what would come next to create the best experience for the client. It took a long time for me to understand that I was reading the collective energy of the room. It also shed light on why teaching a group class was a struggle. The best I can do is trust that everyone is getting what they need.

Yoga teachers repeat the same thing class after class, knowing that the student will only hear the message when they are ready. What teachers say is very different from what students hear.

Most yoga teachers are working out their own personal issues. and I am no different. The true value of yoga is the individual conversation you have with your body on the mat. It is a conversation of the present moment. "Am I tired or energised, am I in pain, and if so, where?" As we practice yoga we experience the blocks and limitations of our lives in movement. I recalled the yoga saying "Body is not stiff, Mind is stiff" from Pattabhi Jois (founder of Ashtanga Yoga).

During the six weeks of lockdown, I was asking those questions daily and again I had to rewrite my truth as to how healthy and balanced I was. Was this another slide down the snake moment? Or was it where the energy rises forth into the true representation of who I am.

My father passed five weeks after his 60th birthday. And he was not the only one in his family to not make it past sixty. The potential of a stroke and a sudden passing was a narrative that I had picked up on and was trying very hard to not buy into. Could I find the courage to see it for what it was – just a story. Or would the fear take me there. I needed to clear it for the past, present and future.

A new client arrived with neck and upper back issues. She reflected an unhealed part of me. I walked away from the session and knew that I wouldn't be sleeping with a pillow (or two) ever again. Why did I do that? As we age it is common to see people walking with their heads bowed. Those extra pillows were cementing the energetics of being defeated by life. I'd already noticed it in my yoga practice that my neck muscles were extremely tight, but to that point hadn't joined the dots. Also, I love doing "plow" pose, which continued the narrative. Instead it was time to open up through the front of the body. It was time to hold my head high.

A colleague offered me her inventory associated with the practice of grounding. 17 years later, I finally followed the advice of the Shaman, and I plugged in to Mother Earth herself.

Remember that spirit animal of mine - the Bear who I had happily popped into hibernation. Well there it was – she was back. Maybe I didn't take up line-dancing, but I was moving with some cosmic flow each morning. And that was enough.

Happiness is the third of the basic human feelings. It comes from a place of "reward". Yes, that overworked word of "gratitude". The hack that sees us being grateful in advance to attract more of what we want into our lives. To be in balance means being grateful for everything, whether it has previously been labelled good or bad. Not what we want or need. To see that everything is a blessing. This creates another level of clearing as things that no longer serve fall away. A natural purge of situations and people as harmony in the present moment becomes the goal.

* * *

A few weeks later while having a consultation with a client (she was in lockdown in Australia), we talked about the book she was long going to write – and how this was the time. My advice was to write it from the present day, rolling back to the beginning - otherwise she would carry the stories forward and nothing would change. It would only be with fresh eyes that she could re-write the narrative and create the healing needed. Immersing self in the story is a powerful way of looking back at the younger you. It creates meaning and insights to the events, and from this comes compassion and forgiveness. Wise words indeed.

Not long after that I opened the computer and begin to immerse myself back in my story. As this book wraps up there is a dialogue about community and support that is swirling around in various guises. Most of this journey I did on my own. It was me and my mat, and a lot of time for self-reflection. Should I have reached out for more support. Absolutely! Time and time again I didn't realise I had a choice.

Turning 60 (and beginning a new decade) may have been the catalyst to unpack these last 10 years. Additionally, the pandemic has been a great leveller. I took my stuff as a personal challenge and kept it very private. Confronting shame is another level of vulnerability needed for the healing journey. I have been nudged to share my learnings in the hope that someone will be able to step out of a difficult place more quickly. Always remembering the saying "Pain is inevitable, suffering is optional".

Shame keeps us in the tightest grip of all. It comes from a place of judgement. A belief that we have done wrong, transgressed in some way. That labelling of human experience as good or bad, rather than seeing the lesson in everything.

And aren't we the harshest critics of ourselves? We have internalised all the "shoulds"; from our family, society, culture, government, religion. This is the patriarchal model we live with – a system that has the infrastructure of control. It takes us out of the universal flow by valuing the head over the heart. The truth is we cannot think ourselves into good health and joy.

We are all going through stuff, we have no idea what personal demons and battles are at play. Compassion is the only answer. My mantra from the teachings of Kyron became: "Show compassion for yourself today, compassion for the situation, and compassion for others."

From this place of compassionate action, we show up from the heart as the best version of ourselves. Beautifully flawed yet engaged in life. Living the best life – which is the healthiest and happiest that is possible in the present moment.

That means finding a connection between what is playing out in the current cycles and relating it to the physical way it is showing up in the body and situations surrounding us. It also means taking responsibility for moving life forward. Having the courage to cast my own lifeline out into the Universe and see what transpires.

Beyond all that – and equally importantly - having the ability to cut myself some slack when it does all spiral downwards (and it continues to do so), use the tools I have learnt to halt the slide, reset then bring myself back into the game. Timing is everything.

* * *

My realisation became that we are all connected. I had done a lot of personal energetic healing work, but I was not immune to the collective fear surfacing. Traditionally empaths and healers were encouraged to put up energy shields as protection. Now we are being asked to increase the vibratory light within to counter the darkness. Dark does not engulf a source of light. Only a switch can turn off the light, and negative emotions (particularly lower vibrations of fear and anger) are the cosmic light switch.

This connectedness includes the state of the planet. Can we look at the level of pollution of the earth without engaging in the discussion of the pollution within our bodies too? The saying from Hermes Trismegistus "as within so without" is on repeat in my mind. Because eventually it is necessary to work the puzzle both ways.

Is it okay:

- To pollute the air, sea and rivers - or ingest chemicals?
- To walk past rubbish on the side of the road, on the beach - or put up with inflammation in the body as arthritis and skin conditions?
- Are our recycling policies encouraging more waste - or do we take personal responsibility for our own health?
- To buy into negativity as entertainment – or live with chronic stress as some "badge of honour"?

Taking the connection to the planet further I explored the elements that make up both our Earth and our Body. The four natural elements are Fire, Earth, Air and Water:

- Fire to burn through inertia and take action.
- Earth to ground into the present moment and provide support.
- Air to initiate change and bring in the required knowledge.
- Water to cleanse and deliver the healing.

My personal favourite is the "Winds of Change", living on a west coast beach provides ample opportunity to feel the changes blowing through. It's a great way to break through moments of "stuck-ness".

I saw how these concepts are present in astrology too. As the sun and moon cycles progress they move through the four elements in rotation, giving us multiple opportunities to work with the differing energies. This connection to the rhythms of nature allows us to access harmony and flow. A state of grace where we drop the need to control and allow situations and insights to occur with divine order.

* * *

Christmas loomed. Did I want to engage with the way things were ? Or was I seeking something different? I knew I was choosing the latter. It was time to turn inwards once again. I began a juice fast. If this book was going to be the deep dive and cathartic process that I envisioned, as well as have clarity and insight; then I needed to come from a space of pure stillness, intuition, and connection to my soul's essence. All the distractions needed to be cast aside.

* * *

What I failed to appreciate was as I immersed myself in the lessons of the past I would be reliving them. Not fully, but enough to recognise them for being an echo of something already dealt with. And when I recently backed the car into another car in the carpark - repeating the experience of my first juice fast - I became very careful and respectful of this part of the journey too.

CHAPTER 40

The Hero's Journey

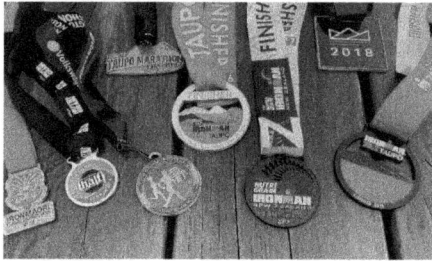

Personal development is the ongoing journey of self-discovery. It doesn't have an end. As one of my best yogi friends told me "How do you know you still have work to do?", "easy answer, as you are still incarnated on earth then there is still work to do!". She finished off with the quip "if you were enlightened you would be gone in a puff of smoke". okay, that brought me back to earth and tamed the ego.

We are all on the hero's journey whether we are consciously aware of it or not. The circumstances of our lives conspire to teach us about ourselves. I use astrology to connect me with the patterns of the cycles at play. Often it feels like a game of balancing multiple spinning plates.

Can I see how things are playing out in these arenas - personal life, relationships, finances, and home?

Is it possible to notice how the same patterns are at play in the periphery, (perhaps at the supermarket checkout), and then maybe with a work colleague, and something similar within the family? Each is an opportunity to inquire as to what the lesson is. The last step is to hold up the mirror and see that we too have the same triggering behaviour – or its exact opposite. That is up to us to balance, to receive the lesson. I found myself repeating the same lessons at increasingly profound levels.

Most people come to the hero's journey via a trigger crisis (usually health related). Most of my crises began after I unwittingly started the process of transformation. Prior to that I did not have the awareness of the opportunity to change. I was stuck in the first half of the resilience equation – enduring what is – and I was very good at it.

I consciously chose to improve my life as I was turning 50. Not in a physical way of Botox and turning back time, or in a material way via new handbags or shoes. What I was pursuing was the deep transformation that radiated from the inside out. Perhaps I wasn't seeking that best version of myself initially, more a chance to set myself up to live my healthiest life as I stepped into the new decade.

And once you start - "let the genie out of the bottle" so to speak there is no going back. In my opinion there is only two ways to progress – medicate or meditate. However, there is always a third option – that decision is to take a hiatus until the clarion call to transform comes again.

* * *

Joseph Campbell's book "The Hero's Journey" describes the concept that we all use as a reference point - knowingly or not. It is the central premise of so many stories, including most of the fairy tales, myths, and legends.

The stages of the hero's journey are:

1. Of being in an ordinary world but feeling dissatisfied. Something is not right yet we can't name the issue.
2. From frustration a challenge or quest is proposed. An opportunity arises that seems imperative yet impractical to pursue.
3. There is an initial refusal of the call. Life is already mapped out and there are valid reasons to decline.
4. Meeting with the mentor. Guidance arrives in the form of people or situations to help end the inertia.
5. Crossing the threshold. Breakthrough occurs and the hero commits to the process.
6. Tests, allies, and enemies. The learning begins as unforeseen circumstances manifest. Discernment is required to see beyond the surface and fully understand.
7. Dealing with the demons. The uncomfortable truth is that we are creating these situations and the solution lies within.
8. The ordeal. Armed with the knowledge that everything is within our control we are required to revisit all beliefs that have led to this moment.
9. Face the fear. New situations arise to test the new belief system.
10. Overcome. Can a more mature response create a different outcome?
11. Rewards. Success comes in a completely different form than prior to the journey.
12. The road back to the ordinary world. Having completed the quest it is time to reengage with life. Bringing forth the wisdom and contributing at a new level.

* * *

Each time I thought I was finished with the journey and it was time to return to the "ordinary world" - the dice rolled again and I found myself being pulled back for another lesson.

At some level I originally wanted to "just be fit". My thinking was that as I got older life would not be an endless list of physical ailments that held me back from enjoying life. At its deepest level it was that calling of "time" of putting other people and situations first. It was time for me. I think I seriously underestimated how low the starting point was.

Equally I didn't plan on devoting my fifties to a seemingly never-ending onslaught of physical challenges and life lessons. It was a bit like how I thought my twenties might well be a mess, but I would enjoy my thirties. Well, half that story was true, my twenties were a mess but then my thirties were another level of difficult. I enjoyed much of my forties and thought that my fifties would be a cruise. Now I'm counting on that cycle repeating and my sixties will be much easier.

* * *

There is much talk in the spiritual circles about connection, community and finding your tribe. That would be amazing! I think this journey is one where you find your tribe for a part of the journey, then there is a need to release the attachment to the group so that you can continue with your growth. Eventually a new tribe arrives. In the interim it is critical to build the relationship with Self - Body and Mind, connecting through Soul to Spirit - so that there is never a feeling of "alone".

* * *

The science of yoga talks of the need to let go of all attachments. Unravelling the story, peeling back the layers - these are what we need to move through as we meditate:

- It starts with the five senses (sight, taste, smell, touch, and hearing).
- It moves into the emotions and feelings.
- Then to conditioning via beliefs (what we have learnt, what we have told ourselves, and what we inherit).
- Lastly to the very nature of our DNA (our concept of what we are capable of in this incarnation).

Once we have let go of the attachments, we are able to connect with the core essence of who we are. The fully manifested self. The Self who chose this time and place to be alive, to have these experiences, learn these lessons, and ultimately to contribute in the ways that are individually appropriate.

My years of international travel had worked to loosen the ropes. I was used to things not being as expected:

- In some countries the on switch is up, and others it's down.
- Is it correct to drive on the left or right side of the road?
- Do we nod our heads to say yes or no.
- Is the working week Monday to Friday, Sunday to Thursday?

Taking this thought of non-attachment to its natural end point - there is the final step where you let go of the "letting go" itself. That is a bit of a mind twist until it becomes clear that it is saying the same as the last stage of the hero's journey. The time when you move out of the journey itself and reintegrate back into life.

Some things I do know: If I hadn't been forced back to Kāpiti I probably wouldn't have stayed in New Zealand. If Ken was still alive, I would not have been focussed on my wellbeing. If I had chosen to care for my mother, I would have been otherwise engaged. If I had found my new tribe it's highly unlikely I would have been so self-absorbed. Was this selfish? Perhaps, in the yoga sutras (my guidebook) the explanation is that the only time being selfish is acceptable is when it is in the pursuit of self-care. If I had not had the 35 Day Detox program on repeat, I would not have identified and cleared "stuff" so relentlessly. So, as difficult as it is to say – these were all the "gifts" of the past decade.

It is comfortable to stay in the familiar; and by now that is the process of examining, clearing, purging, constantly working to improve the version of self that you live with. I believe however, that to be flawed, there is only so much we can do on our own. Eventually it is time to rise above that. We are here for more than ourselves. This is our true purpose, to find devotion to something greater. This is what attracts true joy and happiness from within.

I also want to say a return to "normal life", but in the interim the global pandemic hit and there is no such thing as normal, or even a new normal. It is a whole new world, and we are all trying to find our place in it. We all like certainty, even if we are unhappy, it is uncertainty we find challenging, yet that is exactly where we are supposed to be.

Namaste, the light in me recognises the light in you.

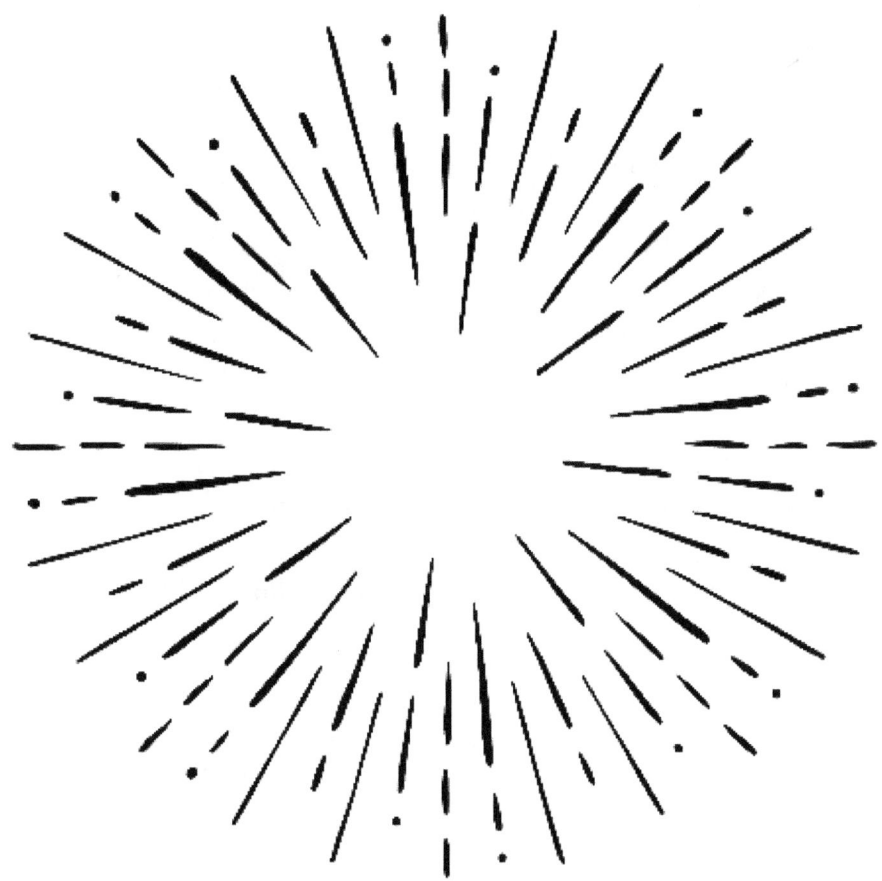

About the Author

Suz Stokes lives in Raumati South, on the Kāpiti Coast, New Zealand with her two dogs, Beau and Jojo. She is the founder of the 35 Day Detox Limited, a health and wellbeing company. The company provides online programs based on the principles of yoga, astrology, numerology and feng shui, healthy whole foods and physical fitness.

Suz is the author of the 2014 Recipe Book – 35 Day Detox, Manifesting Change.

Thank you for taking the time to read my story. I hope it has prompted some recognition of the power you have within you to consciously choose change too.

If the messages within the book have triggered a need to heal, please reach out to the appropriate practitioner for support.

The 35 Day Detox Challenge can be found online at 35daydetox.com

REFERENCES

- Byron Katie 2002 – Loving What Is. Four questions that can change your life.
- Dr Phil McGraw 2002 – Self Matters. Creating your life from the inside out.
- Louise L. Hay 1984 – You can heal your life.
- Dr Robert E. Svoboda 1999 – Ayurveda for women.
- Cuisine Magazines 1990 - 1999
- Edmonds Cookbook
- Sakyong Mipham 2013 – Running with the Mind of Meditation: Lessons for Training Body and Mind.
- Sogyal Rinpoche 1992 – The Tibetan book of living and dying.
- Anodea Judith 2004 – Eastern Body Western Mind. Psychology and the Chakra System as a Path to the Self.
- US Astrologer Molly McCord – www.consciousintuitiveastrology.com
- June Gutmanis 2017 – The Secrets and Practice of Hawaiian Herbal Medicine
- Kyron channelling by Lee Carroll – www.kryon.com
- Joseph Campbell 1990 – The Hero's Journey: Joseph Campbell on His Life and Work.

www.ingramcontent.com/pod-product-compliance
Lightning Source LLC
Chambersburg PA
CBHW072101020426
42334CB00017B/1595